"博学而笃志，切问而近思。"

（《论语》）

博晓古今，可立一家之说；
学贯中西，或成经国之才。

内容简介

　　《当代医学英语视听说教程——健康促进》(第2版)是医学健康学科专业通识教育的新医科英语教材,内容涵盖健康促进领域的基础理论与基础知识,反映当代医学发展"以健康为中心"大趋势与取得的新进展和新成果。通过英语视、听、说、读、写、译融于一体的教学方式,培养医学健康专业素养,发展医学循证思维能力,提升医学健康人文精神,拓展全球视野,为学生进入学科专业学习和自己未来的职业发展做准备。

新医科英语"十四五"全国规划教材

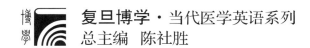

复旦博学·当代医学英语系列
总主编　陈社胜

I
Audio-Visual-Oral English for Medical Purposes
Health Promotion

健康促进

当代医学英语视听说教程 I

（第2版）

主　编　黎　亮　杨克西　李　艳
副主编　戴玥赟　肖　燕　赵　静
编　者（按姓氏笔画排序）

于　洋 (大连医科大学)　　　　曲丽娟 (哈尔滨医科大学)
向　冰 (西南医科大学)　　　　刘黎岗 (成都医学院)
杨克西 (昆明医科大学)　　　　李　艳 (西南医科大学)
肖　燕 (昆明医科大学)　　　　吴　悠 (海南医学院)
宋晓丹 (哈尔滨医科大学)　　　张田仓 (内蒙古医科大学)
张　聪 (大连医科大学)　　　　林滢静雅 (昆明医科大学)
苗　伟 (复旦大学)　　　　　　赵　静 (齐鲁医药学院)
和霁晓 (昆明医科大学)　　　　凌秋虹 (复旦大学)
董妍妍 (大连医科大学)　　　　黎　亮 (成都医学院)
戴玥赟 (山西医科大学)　　　　瞿　平 (哈尔滨医科大学)

英语词汇读录　于　洋 (大连医科大学)
　　　　　　　董妍妍 (大连医科大学)
医学顾问　　马芬芬 (复旦大学附属浦东医院)

复旦大学出版社

序

新时期的大学阶段英语教育为国家发展战略服务，为社会发展服务，为院系专业人才教育和培养服务。医科院校的英语教育目的是为实现人民健康与经济社会协调发展的国家战略，培养合格的各类医药卫生人才，适应和满足新时代医药卫生健康学科专业人才培养的特殊需求。

《当代医学英语视听说教程——健康促进》（第2版）编写以《"健康中国2030"规划纲要》《健康中国行动（2019—2030年）》《大学英语教学指南（2020版）》、教育部《关于一流本科课程建设的实施意见（教高〔2019〕8号）》《普通高等学校健康教育指导纲要》《国民营养计划（2017—2030年）》及国务院《关于加快医学教育创新发展的指导意见（国办发〔2020〕34号）》等文件为依据，以新医科统领新医科英语教育创新发展，为实现以人民健康为中心的国家健康战略服务，为医学院校培养新医科专业人才特殊需求服务，为新医科英语教育创新发展及一流课程建设提供支撑。

作为高等教育重要组成部分的医科教育，目的是培养合格的各类医药卫生人才去推进医药卫生事业发展，促进公众健康水平提升。各类不同人才的培养，要求有不同类型的教育。不言而喻，医学院校的英语教育围绕培养各层次的医药卫生人才展开，是英语教育在医学院校存在的法理基础。但在过去很长的一段时间内，医学院校的英语教育走的是与一般院校英语教育同质化的路径，教学内容缺乏与医药卫生学科专业的联系，缺乏与社会发展联系、缺乏信息量和时代感。显然，这样的教学是无法适应和满足医药卫生学科专业人才培养的特殊需求的。

医学院校的英语教育模式转型应通过更新教育观念、健全教学体系、充实教学内容、创新教学形式，始终面向学生、面向世界、面向未来；使学生为自己职业发展作准备。因此，医学院校的英语教育应是学科性强的专门英语教育。在教育内容上应具有医药卫生专业学科特色，在教学形式上也应避免传统单一的平面化做法。应尽可能应用现代技术，把视、听、说、读、写、译多种教学方式综合于一体，以符合现代学生立体化接受信息和知识的需求。

教之所需，学以致用，是《当代医学英语视听说教程——健康促进》(第2版)的最大特色。教材编写者来自国内医学院校英语教育第一线，既有丰富的英语教学经验，又把握医药卫生学科发展的脉搏，编写了适用于医学院校英语教育的专门用途教材(English for Medical Purpose，EMP)。教材内容突出了医药卫生类学生今后从事职业所需的专业基础知识和基础理论，同时又反映当代医药卫生发展的新理念、新成果，把医学知识获取、创新思维发展、国际视野拓展融入英语教育中，使学生学之有味、学之有获、学之有用。

《当代医学英语视听说教程——健康促进》(第2版)的编者为医学院校英语教育创新和转型发展作出了值得称道的努力，同时也为大学英语教育的可持续发展提供了值得借鉴的范例。

以此，作序致敬。

总主编　陈社胜

2022年11月

前　言

　　《当代医学英语视听说教程——健康促进》(第 2 版)是创新型新医科英语教材,定位于专业通识英语教育,可供医学院校包括预防医学、基础医学、卫生管理、健康教育、医学检验等专业的学生使用。

　　第 2 版编写坚持第 1 版的编写理念,与新医科创新发展同向同行,从内容到形式体现出新医科教育的培养目标。医药卫生类高等院校教育的总体目标,是为推进医药卫生事业发展、促进公众健康水平提升而培养合格的各类医药卫生人才。医学院校的英语教育围绕这一目标展开,是题中应有之义。合格的医药卫生人才,不只是体现在外语水平上,更应体现在专业素养、科学思维、国际视野和人文精神方面。因此,医学院校的英语教育从单一的语言型转变为四位一体的语言习得、专业素质培养、创新思维发展和人文精神提升的综合型教育,是医药卫生类高等院校教育的总体目标之所需,也是新时期社会发展对合格人才之所求。

　　医学的根本目的是促进健康。医学将朝着预言型(predictive)、预防型(preventive)和个性化(personalized)的方向发展,更多地是去管理一个人的健康,而不是去控制一个人的疾病。从事医药卫生事业的合格人才,除了自己身心健康以外,还要运用现代的健康理念和健康科学知识,去促进社会人群的健康。因此,高等医学院校的英语教育从内容到形式都应体现出医学教育的培养目标和当代医学的发展趋势。这样的英语教育有利于学生在英语习得的同时,就能用英语作为工具去获得学科知识和专业信息,有利于学生把所获得的信息和知识转化成智慧,有利于学生面向世界、面向未来,为自己职业发展作准备。

　　《当代医学英语视听说教程——健康促进》(第 2 版)涉及医药卫生合格专业人才必须具备的专业知识核心内容。在学习形式上以视听说为主,着重培养英语听说交流能力。每一项核心内容的视听技能训练包括从单词到句子到篇章的听写、细节辨认、听力笔记、信息补全、简答问题、整体理解;口语交流能力训练项目有文字口译、听译、对话和口述报告等。

　　《当代医学英语视听说教程——健康促进》(第 2 版)也可用于其他高等院校的

健康教育和医学通识教育。教学所需的影像视听资源可通过"i 学 app"获取。教学电子版参考资源可向复旦大学出版社索取。教材中引用的音视频资料,来源于 ABC News,NBC Health News,CBS 和 VOA Health Report 等公共英语媒体。编者对资料来源的媒体机构和作者深表感谢。编者同样感谢复旦大学出版社为推动大学英语教育转型和创新作出的努力。本教材编写还得到了相关医学院校主管大学外语教育领导的支持和帮助,编者在此一并致谢。

编者

2022 年 11 月

Contents

Unit 3   Sleep and Health   19

Overview

Unit 4   Physical Exercise   28

Overview

Unit 5   Weight Control 37

Overview

Unit 8 Environment and Health 66

Overview

Unit 9 Stress Management 75

Overview

Unit 10   Coping with Depression   84

Overview

Unit 11   First Aid   94

Overview

Unit 12 Preventing Epidemics 103

Overview

Unit 13 Screening and Checkup 113

Overview

General Introduction

The WHO's 1986 Ottawa Charter for Health Promotion and then the 2005 Bangkok Charter for Health Promotion in a Globalized World defines health promotion as "the process of enabling people to increase control over their health and its determinants, and thereby improve their health".

Health promotion involves public policy that addresses health determinants such as income, housing, food security, employment, and quality working conditions. More recent work has used the term Health in All Policies to refer to the actions that incorporate health into all public policies.

Health promotion is aligned with health equity and can be a focus of non-governmental organizations (NGOs) dedicated to social justice or human rights. Health literacy can be developed in schools, while aspects of health promotion such as breastfeeding promotion can depend on laws and rules of public spaces. One of the Ottawa Charter Health Promotion Action items is infusing prevention into all sectors of society, to that end, it is seen in preventive healthcare rather than a treatment and curative care focused medical model.

There is a tendency among some public health officials, governments, and the medical industrial complex to reduce health promotion to just developing personal skills, also known as health education and social marketing focused on changing behavioral risk factors. However, recent evidence suggests that attitudes about public health policies are less about personal abilities or health messaging than about individuals' philosophical beliefs about morality, politics, and science.

In the higher education setting, the process of health promotion is applied within a post-secondary academic environments to increase health and wellbeing. The process needs professionals to engage in all five WHO Ottawa

Charter Health Promotion Actions and particularly reorient all the sectors of a college campus towards evidence-based prevention, utilizing a public health/population health/community health model. Health promotion requires a coordinated effort in all five Actions:

1. Building healthy public policy

2. Creating supportive environments

3. Strengthening community action

4. Developing personal skills

5. Re-orienting all service sectors toward prevention of illness and promotion of health

The basic strategies for health promotion are prioritized as:

Advocate: Health is a resource for social and developmental means, thus the dimensions that affect these factors must be changed to encourage health.

Enable: Health equity must be reached where individuals must become empowered to control the determinants that affect their health, such that they are able to reach the highest attainable quality of life.

Mediation: Health promotion cannot be achieved by the health sector alone; rather its success will depend on the collaboration of all sectors of government (social, economic, etc.) as well as independent organizations (media, industry, universities, etc.).

Healthy Living

Overview

The World Health Organization (WHO) defined health in its broader sense in 1946 as "a state of complete physical, mental, and social well-being and not merely the absence of disease or infirmity."

The term "healthy" is widely used in the context of many types of non-living organizations and their impacts for the benefit of humans, such as in the sense of healthy communities, healthy cities or healthy environments. In addition to health-care interventions and a person's surroundings, a number of other factors are known to influence the health status of individuals, including their background, lifestyle, and economic and social conditions; these are referred to as "determinants of health".

Numerous studies suggest that people can improve their health via exercise, enough sleep, maintaining a healthy body weight, limiting alcohol use, and avoiding smoking.

Section A   Pre-audio-visual Tasks

Task 1   Glossary Work

Get familiar with the following words and expressions by listening to and reading them. Then match the meaning description or synonym with a proper word or expression in the glossary list.

impact /ˈɪmpækt/	n.	影响；冲击	
obesity /əʊˈbɪsətɪ/	n.	肥胖，肥胖症	
waist-hip /weɪst hɪp/	adj.	腰臀的	
modification /ˌmɒdɪfɪˈkeɪʃn/	n.	改变；变形；变更；修正	
diabetes /ˌdaɪəˈbiːtiːz/	n.	糖尿病	
stroke /strəʊk/	n.	卒中，中风	
locale /ləʊˈkɑːl/	n.	场所或地点	
disorder /dɪsˈɔːdə(r)/	n.	（身心）失调；不适；病	
disability /ˌdɪsəˈbɪlətɪ/	n.	残疾；无能	
medication /ˌmedɪˈkeɪʃn/	n.	药物，药剂；药物治疗	
reinforce /ˌriːɪnˈfɔːs/	v.	加强	
kick /kɪk/	v.	戒除	
automate /ˈɔːtəmeɪt/	v.	使自动化	
whopping /ˈwɒpɪŋ/	a.	不平常的；巨大的；庞大的	
sedentary /ˈsednterɪ/	adj.	久坐不活动的	
rinse /rɪns/	v.	冲洗；冲掉	
benign /bɪˈnaɪn/	adj.	（肿瘤）良性的；温和的	
asthma /ˈæzmə/	n.	哮喘；气喘	
friction /ˈfrɪkʃn/	n.	摩擦；摩擦力；冲突；不和	
deliberate /dɪˈlɪbərət/	adj.	蓄意的；小心翼翼的	
cardiovascular /ˌkɑːdɪəʊˈvæskjələ(r)/	adj.	心血管的	
add up		言之有理；加起来得到理想的结果	
life expectancy		期望寿命，平均寿命	
body mass index		身体质量指数，体重指数	
cut short		缩短；剪短；截断	
junk food		垃圾食品；无营养食品	
premature death		过早死亡	
in shape		处于良好状况	
blood clots		血凝块	
keep . . . at bay		防止……发生	

1. inability to pursue an occupation because of physical or mental impairment

2. the average number of years that a person or animal can expect to live

   _____

3. an abnormal physical or mental condition

   _____

4. in good physical condition

   _____

5. food that is of little nutritional value and often high in fat, sugar, and calories

   _____

6. a serious illness caused when a blood vessel in your brain suddenly breaks or is blocked

   _____

7. a substance used in treating disease or relieving pain; the act or process of treating a person or disease with medicine

   _____

8. the place where something happens

   _____

9. characterized by much sitting and little physical exercise

   _____

10. a medical condition in which excess body fat has accumulated to the extent that it may have an adverse effect on health

    _____

11. to strengthen or support (an object or substance), especially with additional material

    _____

12. a change in something; the act or process of changing parts of something

    _____

13. a powerful or major influence or effect; the act or force of one thing hitting another

    _____

14. a measurement that shows the amount of fat in your body and that is based on your weight and height

    _____

15. a variable disorder of carbohydrate metabolism usually characterized by inadequate secretion or utilization of insulin, by excessive urine production, by excessive amounts of sugar in the blood and urine, and by thirst, hunger, and loss of weight

    _____

Section B   Audio-visual Tasks

Task 2   Spot Dictation

Listen to a passage twice and while listening, you are to put the missing words in each numbered blank according to what you hear.

Lifestyle choices such as diet and exercise can have a big impact on health. The (1) _____ is full of studies about the effect of various lifestyle factors, but relatively few studies look at the combined influence of multiple factors, and almost all of them were done in Western countries.

Now, a large new study of Chinese women (2) _____ of the healthy lifestyle choices can really add up. The research considers factors such as obesity and (3) _____ second-hand smoke. Numerous studies have worked the link between specific lifestyle factors such as exercise and diet, and risks of disease and death, but much less research has been done (4) _____ _____ of multiple unhealthy life style choices. Now a large study in women in Shanghai has found a (5) _____ between a healthy lifestyle in general and a lower death rate, over an average of nine years.

Dr. Wei Zheng of Vanderbilt University is the (6) _____ of the new study, which also included researchers from the Shanghai Cancer Institute and America's National Cancer Institute.

In this study, some (7) _____ Chinese women were each given a healthy lifestyle score based on body mass index, waist-hip ratio, exercise, diet, and whether her husband smoked. The women were non-smokers and did not (8) _____ regularly.

Zheng says the research suggests that a longer and healthier life (9) _____ _____ by just a better diet or more exercise or other single lifestyle factor alone.

"So the message from this study is that we need to encourage (10) _____ _____ of multiple lifestyle factors for disease prevention."

Task 3   Note-taking

Listen to the passage "Life Expectancy and Lifestyle Choices" twice. While listening, you are to take notes according to the cues given below.

1. Life expectancy in wealthy nations increased in the 20th century:

_____

2. Examples of bad habits:

_____

3. Bad habits increase the risk for:

_____

4. What researchers wanted to find out:

_____

5. The purpose of programs planned by public health officials:

_____

Task 4   Sentence Dictation

Listen to each sentence, repeat it aloud, listen to it again, and then write down the whole sentence in the space provided.

1. _____
   _____

2. _____
   _____

3. _____
   _____

4. _____
   _____

5. _____
   _____

Task 5   Recognizing Details

Watch the video clip "Your Daily Routine Is Ruining Your Health" twice and decide whether each of the statements below is TRUE (T) *or* FALSE (F).

_____ 1. Smoking, drinking and bingeing on junk food are some benign daily routines.

_____ 2. You may actually feel more tired after getting 8 hours of sleep each night.

_____ 3. Some dentists say that rinsing does not offer your teeth a protective fluorine coating.

_____ 4. Showering every day using super-hot water with hard soaps is not a good routine.

_____ 5. It is not a bad routine to do house cleaning right when you get home from work.

_____ 6. Some studies suggest household cleaning may help reduce high blood pressure.

_____ 7. You could ask somebody else to pick up some of the housework to avoid some health problems.

Task 6　Overall Comprehension

Watch the video clip "The Secret of Habits" twice and choose the best answer to each of the questions below.

1. According to Dr. Windy, a habit is _____.
　　A. an act of conscious choices　　　　B. something relying on willpower
　　C. a goal of self-training　　　　　　D. what we do every single day
2. Which of the following is not mentioned as a good habitual behavior?
　　A. Eating better.　　　　　　　　　B. Putting phone down.
　　C. Reading books.　　　　　　　　　D. Exercising more.
3. To create a good behavior, you need to do all of the following EXCEPT _____.
　　A. rely on willpower　　　　　　　　B. find something you enjoy
　　C. do it and repeat it　　　　　　　D. break some bad habits
4. According to Dr. Windy, you form a habit if you _____.
　　A. remove some friction　　　　　　B. feel some sort of enjoyment
　　C. do something consciously　　　　D. have a strong determination
5. Even for an act to become a simple habit you have to _____.
　　A. repeat it deliberately　　　　　　B. find a substitute for it
　　C. focus on the outcome　　　　　　D. do something simple first

Section C　Oral Tasks

Task 7　Listening & Interpretation

Listen to each sentence twice and interpret it into Chinese.

1. _____

_____

2. _____

_____

3. _____

_____

4. _____

_____

5. _____

_____

Task 8　Dialogue & Conversation

Make dialogues and conversations , using the Chinese below as cues .

A: 你对生活方式与健康的关系怎么看?

B: 这两者的关系很密切。健康的生活方式会增进健康,不良的生活方式有损健康。

A: 很多人没有意识到不良的生活方式是影响健康的重大危险因素。

B: 情况确实如此。据你观察,你周围的人群中有哪些不健康的生活方式选择?

A: 有不少,如过量饮食、吃垃圾食品、吸烟、酗酒、缺睡眠、少运动,等等。

B: 这些不健康的生活方式选择与哪些健康问题相联系?

A: 许多新的研究表明,生活方式不健康的人群有更高的肥胖症、卒中、糖尿病和过早死亡的风险。当然,风险还不止这些。

B: 你所说的使我想起一句话很有道理:你的健康是你选择的结果。

A: 有健康才有高的生活质量,才有快乐的人生。

B: 我很同意你的看法。健康不是天生的,健康不仅是意识,更是主动行动的结果。

Task 9   Discussion or Oral Presentation

Discuss briefly in a pair-group or make a 2-minute oral presentation based on the following questions.

1. What does lifestyle refer to?
2. What is the relationship between lifestyle and health?
3. What are examples of an unhealthy lifestyle?
4. What do you think of your own lifestyle?
5. What can you do to improve your lifestyle?

Section D   Follow-up Reading

Task 10   Reading Comprehension

Read the passage and fill in each blank with a proper phrase or sentence given in the box.

In the 20th century, life expectancy in wealthy nations increased by as much as 30 years. Average life expectancy for Americans is 78.

But doctors are seeing people __1__, like eating too much or eating too much junk food, exercising too little and smoking cigarettes. These habits increase the risk for cancer, diabetes, heart disease and stroke.

Researchers at Harvard University and the University of Washington wanted to __2__. The researchers broke down the data into race, income and locale and they found even greater differences. Middle-income whites have the best blood pressure. But Asian-Americans __3__.

The researchers found a 14-year difference in life expectancy between Asian-American and African-American men who can expect to live an average of 67 years.

African-American women __4__ because of their high rates of obesity. People battling excess weight have higher rates of disability, diabetes and heart disease — disorders that make them sicker at younger ages and dependent on medications for many years.

The researchers say public health officials could use the study to plan programs that will __5__.

_____ 1.	A.	help people make better lifestyle choices
_____ 2.	B.	have fewer bad habits and the best health
_____ 3.	C.	are another group with low life expectancy
_____ 4.	D.	adopt bad habits that can cut their lives short
_____ 5.	E.	are among groups with highest life expectancy
	F.	help them educe the risk for cardiovascular diseases
	G.	find out how many years are lost with these lifestyle choices

Healthy Diet

Overview

A healthy diet is one that helps maintain or improve health. It is important for the prevention of many chronic diseases such as obesity, heart disease, diabetes, and cancer. A healthy diet involves consuming appropriate amounts all of the food groups, including an adequate amount of water. Nutrients can be obtained from many different foods, so there are a wide variety of healthy diets.

The World Health Organization estimates that 2.7 million deaths are attributable to a diet low in fruit and vegetable every year. Globally it is estimated to cause about 19% of gastrointestinal cancer, 31% of ischemic (缺血性的) heart disease, and 11% of strokes. Thus making it one of the leading preventable causes of death worldwide.

It is known that the experiences we have in childhood relating to consumption of food affect our perspective on food consumption in later life. From this, we are able to determine our limits of how much we will eat, as well as foods we will not eat.

Indeed, ideas of what counts as "healthy eating" have varied in different times and places, according to scientific advances in the field of nutrition, cultural fashions, or personal considerations.

Section A   Pre-audio-visual Tasks

Task 1   Glossary Work

Get familiar with the following words and expressions by listening to and reading them . Then complete each of the sentences with a proper word from the list .

serving /ˈsɜːvɪŋ/ *n .*	一人份
dietary /ˈdaɪətərɪ/ *adj .*	饮食的;规定饮食的
lycopene /ˈlaɪkəpiːn/ *n .*	番茄红素
spinach /ˈspɪnɪtʃ/ *n .*	菠菜
fetus /ˈfiːtəs/ *n .*	胎儿
homocystine /həʊməʊˈsɪstiːn/ *n .*	高胱氨酸
broccoli /ˈbrɒkəlɪ/ *n .*	花椰菜,西兰花
oat /əʊt/ *n .*	燕麦;麦片粥
blockage /ˈblɒkɪdʒ/ *n .*	堵塞
artery /ˈɑːtərɪ/ *n .*	动脉
Alzheimer's disease /ˈæltshaɪməzdɪˈziːz/ *n .*	阿尔茨海默病
salmon /ˈsæmən/ *n .*	鲑鱼,大马哈鱼
herring /ˈherɪŋ/ *n .*	鲱鱼
mackerel /ˈmækrəl/ *n .*	鲭鱼
bluefish /ˈbluːfɪʃ/ *n .*	蓝鱼,跳鱼
cholesterol /kəˈlestərɒl/ *n .*	胆固醇
blueberries /ˈbluːberɪz/ *n .*	蓝莓
bladder /ˈblædə(r)/ *n .*	膀胱;囊状物
colorectal /kəʊləˈrektəl/ *adj .*	结直肠的
saturated /ˈsætʃəreɪtɪd/ *adj .*	饱和的
variability /verɪəˈbɪlətɪ/ *n .*	可变性;易变性
consume /kənˈsjuːm/ *v .*	消费
cutback /ˈkʌtbæk/ *n .*	减少;削减
villain /ˈvɪlən/ *n .*	坏人,恶棍,罪犯
crusade /kruːˈseɪd/ *n .*	改革运动
trans fat	反式脂肪
digestive system	消化系统
folic acid	叶酸
fatty acid	脂肪酸
Mediterranean diet	地中海饮食

1. Both groups had the same rates of heart disease and _____ cancer.

2. Their high living standards cause their present population to _____ 25 percent of the world's oil.

3. The dark green vegetable spinach contains _____ that prevents problems in developing fetuses.

4. Having too much _____ in your blood can lead to serious medical problems such as heart attacks and strokes.

5. Fish that contain omega 3 fatty acids help prevent _____ in the arteries.

6. _____ fats that are found in foods such as meat and butter are not easily processed by the body.

7. He is opposed to further _____ in healthcare spending.

8. Patients were asked to empty their _____ before going to bed.

9. I hope this article will offer insight into the risks, benefits, and indications for use of this _____ therapy.

10. Bodybuilders should consume at least eight _____ of fruit and vegetables a day.

11. Poorly controlled asthma can lead to serious medical problems for pregnant women and their _____.

12. As blood travels around the body in _____ and veins, it is under pressure.

13. They remind Americans to eat more whole grains and fruits and vegetables, while limiting consumption of _____ and alcohol.

14. We all need to support the _____ against corruption.

15. The disease is more than just a disorder of the _____ and affects the whole body.

Section B   Audio-visual Tasks

Task 2   Spot Dictation

Listen to a passage twice and while listening, you are to put the missing words in each numbered blank according to what you hear.

For years, medical experts have thought that a diet that is low in fat helps reduce the risk of cancer and heart disease. Researchers with America's National Institutes of Health created a study to (1) _____. It is one of the largest studies ever done on this subject. The researchers studied the health of almost (2) _____ women for eight years. These women were between the ages of 50 and 79 years.

The women in one group reduced the fat in their diet to 20 percent of their total daily food supply. They also increased their (3) _____ of vegetables, fruits and grains. Another group of women did not make any (4) _____ __. The researchers compared the two groups.

The results of the study show the different diets had little effect on the health of the women. Both groups had the same rates of heart disease and (5) _____ ____. The researchers said the women who followed the low-fat diet might have less risk of breast cancer. But the difference was so small that it is not considered important.

Experts say the results are important for both men and women. (6) _____ _____ of the study fear many people will think that diet is not important. Other studies have shown that a healthful diet is still important, but so are other choices. For example, exercising, (7) _____, and keeping a normal body weight are also necessary for good health.

Other experts noted the study (8) _____ reducing total fat instead of the kinds of fats that are not healthful. For example, fats in some foods like fish and nuts are considered good for human health. Unhealthful fats include saturated and (9) _____. The study did not note differences between these two kinds of fat.

Experts also said that dietary changes might need to begin earlier in life to have a greater (10) _____ disease and cancer prevention.

Task 3   Short Answer Questions

Listen to the passage "Food and Health" twice. While listening, you are to give an answer as short as possible to each of the questions below.

1. What do many substances in foods help to do?

_____

2. What problems does folic acid in the dark green vegetables help prevent?

3. What do oats help to improve in addition to lowering blood pressure?

4. How may garlic help protect the heart?

5. What health problems have blueberries been shown to help protect against?

Task 4   Sentence Dictation

Listen to each sentence, repeat it aloud, listen to it again, and then write down the whole sentence in the space provided.

1. _____

2. _____

3. _____

4. _____

5. _____

Task 5   Recognizing Details

Watch the video clip "The Mediterranean Diet" twice and decide whether each of the statements below is TRUE (T) *or* FALSE (F).

_____ 1. Every year 40 million Americans make a pledge to improve how they eat.

_____ 2. 25 top nutritionists, physicians, and researchers have been convened to rank the diets based on eight different categories.

_____ 3. The Mediterranean diet ranked number one in a tie with a DASH diet for the first time.

_____ 4. The DASH diet aims to prevent and lower high blood pressure.

_____ 5. We need vitamin as a source of energy.

_____ 6. Fats in our diet help us to absorb those vitamins.

_____ 7. Healthy diets are fairly low in protein and they all pretty much minimize or avoid processed foods.

Task 6　Overall Comprehension

Watch the video clip "Cutting Salt Consumption" twice and choose the best answer to each of the questions below.

1. It is mentioned in the video that most of the salt problem is _____.

   A. hidden salt
   B. health risks
   C. heart attacks
   D. high blood pressure

2. Salt is a very serious problem _____.

   A. for every American
   B. causing major diseases
   C. in food supply in the U.S.
   D. caused by food manufacturers

3. The FDA is doing all of the following EXCEPT _____.

   A. considering ways to cut salt consumption
   B. working with food manufacturers
   C. setting new lower salt standards
   D. limiting salt to 2300 milligrams a day

4. According to the CDC, only small percentage of the salt Americans consume comes from _____.

   A. home-cooked food
   B. processed food
   C. restaurant food
   D. packaged food

5. New York City has launched an anti-salt crusade to _____.

   A. eliminate possible harms caused by too much salt
   B. cut salt levels by 25% over the next five years
   C. reduce the health risks of unhealthy eating
   D. educate its residents about the risks of salt

Section C Oral Tasks

Task 7   Listening & Interpretation

Listen to each sentence twice and interpret each it Chinese.

1. _____

_____

2. _____

_____

3. _____

_____

4. _____

_____

5. _____

_____

Task 8   Dialogue & Conversation

Make dialogues and conversations, using the Chinese below as cues.

A: 现在民众对饮食影响健康的作用的认识在不断提高。

B: 是的。不过,很多人对健康饮食的概念仍然不清楚,也不知道怎样的饮食才是健康的饮食。

A: 健康的饮食是指一种有助于维持或改善整体健康的饮食。比如,地中海饮食就是一种健康饮食。

B: 是不是健康的饮食还应含有水果、蔬菜和全谷物,很少或不包括加工食品?

A: 是的。在健康饮食方面,世界卫生组织提出了5项建议,包括限制脂肪摄入,避免反式脂肪,限制每日盐和糖的摄入等。

B: 不健康饮食会对个人健康有哪些不利的影响?

A: 不健康的饮食是许多慢性病的一个主要风险因素,包括高血压、高胆固醇、糖尿病、心血管疾病和癌症等。

B: 不健康饮食危害有这么多啊!

A：世界卫生组织估计，21世纪每年有270万人死于水果和蔬菜饮食不足。

B：看来饮食改变可能需要在生活中更早地开始，才能对疾病预防有更大的影响。

Task 9   Discussion or Oral Presentation

Discuss briefly in a pair-group or make a 2-minute oral presentation based on the following questions.

1. What are your favorite foods? Why do you think your favorite foods are healthy or unhealthy?
2. Why is a low-fat diet/low-salt diet beneficial to our health?
3. What substances in foods are thought to have effects beneficial to health?
4. What are obstacles to adopting a healthy eating habit?
5. What can health institutions do to overcome obstacles to a healthy diet?

Section D   Follow-up Reading

Task 10   Reading Comprehension

Read the passage and complete each statement with a proper phrase or sentence given in the box.

Most Americans, nine out of every ten, consume too much salt and face the health risks that go along with that. The problem is, most of it is hidden salt, added to food before it ever reaches your plate. But now there's a move to cutback.

In the battle against high blood pressure, heart attacks and strokes, health experts say too much salt has emerged as a clear villain. "Salt is a very serious problem in our food supply. It is a major cause of disease in this country," said Margaret Hamburg, FDA commissioner.

Now for the first time, the FDA is considering ways to cut salt consumption by working with food manufacturers to set new lower salt standards. Dietary guidelines generally call for limiting salt to 2,300 milligrams a day, a little more than one teaspoon of salt. But Americans regularly consume 50% more, even double that, everyday. Registered dietitian Colleen Gerg says salt or sodium seems to be in every can, jar, bottle and box in the grocery store. "If you were to eat this one whole can of soup, you would be consuming 2,300 milligrams of sodium, exactly the amount that you should get in an entire day," Gerg said.

The CDC reports that only 5% of the salt that we consume comes from home cooking, 6% comes from the salt we add while eating. Most of the salt or sodium we eat comes from packaged, processed, store-bought and restaurant food.

That morning bacon, egg and cheese biscuit on the way to work can have up to 1360 mg of salt. A portion of cheese pizza, anywhere from 400 to 800 mg. French fries: 270 to 960 mg, depending on the restaurant. And that cheeseburger, 750 to 970 mg of salt. New York City has already launched an anti-salt crusade pushing food manufacturers and restaurants to cut salt levels by 25% over the next five years.

Now the FDA is looking at gradually cutting salt levels over the coming decade. The hope is that by cutting down on the sodium content over the next ten years, Americans won't notice any difference in taste. "We have conditioned our pallets to want this much sodium in our food, and you can decondition your pallet in the same way by eating a lot less processed food and eating fresh whole foods," Gerg said.

A new emphasis is on salt awareness and healthy eating.

1. Most Americans consume too much salt, most of which _____.
2. According to experts, too much salt _____.
3. Dietary guidelines generally call for limiting salt to 2,300 milligrams a day, but Americans _____.
4. According to the CDC report, most of the salt we eat _____.
5. The FDA is considering gradually cutting salt levels over the coming decade and the emphasis _____.

A. consume lot less processed food

B. is a major cause of disease in the U.S.

C. regularly consume more than that everyday

D. is added to food before it ever reaches your plate

E. is on the awareness of health risks associated with it

F. comes from packaged, processed, and restaurant food

G. is launching an anti-salt crusade throughout the country

Sleep and Health

Overview

Sleep is a natural state of rest characterized by reduced body movement and decreased awareness of surroundings. While the exact purpose of sleep remains a mystery, sleep researchers have made enormous strides in understanding how sleep occurs in humans and other animals, and the nature of sleep disorders.

Researches show that seven to nine hours of sleep for adult humans is optimal (最优的) and that sufficient sleep benefits alertness(清醒), memory, problem solving, and overall health, as well as reducing the risk of accidents.

Researchers have found that lack of sleep can more than double the risk of death from cardiovascular(心血管的) disease, but that too much sleep can also double the risk of death. Furthermore, sleep difficulties are closely associated with psychiatric(精神病的) disorders such as depression. Up to 90% of patients with depression are found to have sleep difficulties.

Sleep debt is the effect of not getting enough rest and sleep; a large debt causes mental, emotional, and physical fatigue. It is unclear why a lack of sleep causes irritability(易怒); however, theories are emerging that suggest if the body produces insufficient cortisol during deep sleep, it can have negative effects on the alertness and emotions of a person during the day.

In both children and adults, short sleep duration is associated with an increased risk of obesity, with various studies reporting an increased risk of 45 − 55%. Other aspects of sleep health have been associated with obesity, including daytime napping, sleep timing，the variability of sleep timing, and low sleep efficiency.

Section A Pre-audio-visual Tasks

Task 1 Glossary Work

Get familiar with the following words and expressions by listening to and reading them. Then match the meaning description or synonym with a proper word or expression in the glossary list.

target /ˈtɑːgɪt/ *v*.	把……作为目标
astronaut /ˈæstrənɔːt/ *n*.	宇航员
tiredness /ˈtaɪədnəs/ *n*.	疲劳,疲倦
emotion /ɪˈməʊʃn/ *n*.	情感;情绪
mistakenly /mɪˈsteɪkənlɪ/ *adv*.	错误地;曲解地
identify /aɪˈdentɪfaɪ/ *v*.	确定;认同
hyperactivity /ˌhaɪpərækˈtɪvətɪ/ *n*.	极度活跃;活动过度
tension /ˈtenʃn/ *n*.	紧张;焦虑;冲突
urge /ɜːdʒ/ *v*.	催促;驱使
briefly /ˈbriːflɪ/ *adv*.	短暂地;简略地
effectiveness /ɪfekˈtɪvnɪs/ *n*.	效力
wage /weɪdʒ/ *v*.	进行;开展
sleep-deprived /sliːp dɪˈpraɪvd/ *adj*.	睡眠不足的
transportation /ˌtrænspɔːˈteɪʃn/ *n*.	运输
adopt /əˈdɒpt/ *v*.	采取;收养
exhaustion /ɪgˈzɔːstʃən/ *n*.	精疲力竭;耗尽
relief /rɪˈliːf/ *n*.	减轻;宽慰;解脱
consequence /ˈkɒnsɪkwens/ *n*.	结果;重要性
previously /ˈpriːvɪəslɪ/ *adv*.	先前
dramatically /drəˈmætɪklɪ/ *adv*.	显著地;引人注目地
inflammation /ˌɪnfləˈmeɪʃən/ *n*.	发炎;炎症
dysregulation /diːzregjʊˈleɪʃn/ *n*.	失调
affect /əˈfekt/ *v*.	影响;感染
concerning /kənˈsɜːnɪŋ/ *prep*.	关于;就……而言
a big chunk of	大量的

delivery business	运输;快递业
all sorts of	各种各样的
car crash	车祸
beat the clock	提前完成任务
The American Academy of Pediatrics	美国儿科学会

1. to aim an attack at a particular object, place, or person _____

2. to recognize and correctly name someone or something _____

3. wrongly; in a mistaken way _____

4. abnormality or impairment in the regulation of a metabolic, physiological, or psychological process _____

5. to finish something or succeed before time is up _____

6. a result or effect, typically one that is unwelcome or unpleasant _____

7. to accept or to form a relationship with another person (as to take a child as one's own) _____

8. extreme tiredness; fatigue _____

9. a localized physical condition in which part of the body becomes reddened, swollen, hot, and often painful, especially as a reaction to injury or infection

_____

10. before; at an earlier time; in the past; antecedently _____

11. a feeling of reassurance and relaxation following release from anxiety or distress _____

12. to influence; move someone (emotionally); attack (of a disease) _____

13. regarding; about _____

14. by a strikingly large amount or to a strikingly large extent; greatly _____

15. a feeling of nervousness before an important or difficult event _____

Section B Audio-visual Tasks

Task 2   Spot Dictation

Listen to a passage twice and while listening, you are to put the missing words in each numbered blank according to what you hear.

For many years, officials of the National Institutes of Health have told Americans that they need to get enough sleep to stay healthy and (1) _____ .

In the past, the NIH targeted special groups, like drivers, soldiers and astronauts. Now, health officials have (2) _____ to urge children to get enough sleep. The officials say children need at least 9 hours of sleep every night. They say research shows that children who get this much sleep perform better in school, (3) _____ and are less likely to become too fat.

Studies show that lack of sleep (4) _____ and problems with clear thinking. People who do not get enough sleep become angry easily and have trouble (5) _____ .

Among children, problems that result from lack of sleep often (6) _____ more serious disorders. Unlike adults, tired children seem to have endless energy. Some doctors mistakenly identify this (7) _____ .

Experts say many American teenagers are not getting enough sleep. Teenagers (8) _____ for several reasons, including schoolwork, after school activities and late-night fun.

The American Academy of Pediatrics (9) _____ who treat children. It notes that many sleep disorders first develop in childhood. It says doctors often do not (10) _____ until years later.

Task 3　Note-taking

Listen to the passage "Take a Nap" twice. While listening, you are to take notes according to the cues given below.

1. Research found persons who sleep for a few minutes during the day were:

_____

2. How naps might improve health for working men:

_____

3. Some companies believe that letting workers rest briefly in their office reduces:

_____

4. In addition to providing extra energy, a nap can:

5. Optimal length of a nap according to experts:

_____

Task 4   Sentence Dictation

Listen to each sentence, repeat it aloud, listen to it again, and then write down the whole sentence in the space provided.

1. _____

   _____

2. _____

   _____

3. _____

   _____

4. _____

   _____

5. _____

   _____

Task 5   Recognizing Details

Watch the video clip "Sleep Deprivation Dangerous to Health" twice and decide whether each of the statements below is TRUE (T) *or* FALSE (F).

_____ 1. A big chunk of the American work force, 41 million people get far too enough sleep.

_____ 2. Many of us are losing the struggle of getting enough sleep.

_____ 3. About two thirds of working adults get six or fewer hours every day of sleep.

_____ 4. Among health care workers, over half said they don't sleep enough.

_____ 5. Many studies have shown a lack of sleep increases the risk for heart disease, obesity and diabetes.

_____ 6. The CDC says people who work nights should adopt a special sleep routine.

_____ 7. The battle of getting enough sleep is waged by millions of Americans with relief in sight.

Task 6   Overall Comprehension

Watch the video clip "Sleep Deprivation and Stroke Risk" twice and choose the best answer to each of the questions below.

1. The health news is mainly about _____ .

    A. a rare commodity in many homes across the U.S.

    B. the real consequences for sleep-deprived people

    C. the dysregulation in blood pressure

    D. contributing factors to sleep deprivation

2. Which of the following is NOT mentioned as a consequence of too little sleep?

    A. Dramatically increased risks of stroke.

    B. Dysregulation in blood pressure.

    C. Increased blood flow to the brain.

    D. Increased inflammation in the body.

3. Which of the following statements is NOT true of stroke?

    A. It is a contributing factor to sleep deprivation.

    B. It is the fourth leading cause of death in the U.S.

    C. It's more common in people with high blood pressure.

    D. It occurs when the blood flow to the brain is interrupted.

4. What makes the new research more concerning?

    A. More than 56,000 people involved were not overweight.

    B. More than 56,000 people were more likely to suffer a stroke.

    C. More than 56,000 people got less than six hours of sleep at night.

    D. More than 56,000 people stopped all those activities earlier in the night.

5. A worrying conclusion is that _____ .

    A. not smoking and getting some fresh air are all we need to do

    B. reducing your weight may contribute to getting enough sleep

    C. dysregulation in blood pressure is caused by sleep loss

    D. sleep has to be on the list of how we keep ourselves healthy

Section C   Oral Tasks

Task 7   Listening & Interpretation

Listen to each sentence twice and interpret it into Chinese.

1. _____

   _____

2. _____

   _____

3. _____

   _____

4. _____

   _____

5. _____

   _____

Task 8   Dialogue & Conversation

Make dialogues and conversations, using the Chinese below as cues.

A：睡眠与健康有密切的联系。不幸的是,不少人不把睡眠当回事。

B：是啊,健康生活的一部分就是要有充足的睡眠。你每晚要睡多少时间呢?

A：我通常睡 7～8 小时,偶尔睡 6 小时,但从不熬夜。

B：看来你的睡眠习惯不错。睡眠时间多少,会随一些因素而有所不同,但孩子们每晚应睡足 9 小时。

A：充足的睡眠有助于他们在学校表现得更好,避免意外事故的发生和减少肥胖的概率。

B：充足的睡眠还带来其他健康好处,如减少患心脏病和卒中的风险。

A：有人认为,可以用均衡饮食和适当运动来弥补睡眠的不足。你怎么看?

B：虽然适当的运动、均衡饮食和充足的睡眠是国际社会公认的 3 项健康标准,但它们对健康的作用是不同的,也是无可替代的。

A：所以，经常以少睡来换取其他东西，从长远来看是得不偿失的。难道还有比健康更重要的东西吗？

B：关注睡眠，就是关注健康。因睡眠不足导致的健康问题是健康生活中不容忽视的。

Task 9   Discussion or Oral Presentation

Discuss briefly in a pair-group or make a 2-minute oral presentation based on the following questions.

1. How many hours of sleep are considered to be healthy for adults?
2. What are the possible consequences of a large "sleep debt"?
3. Do you support the idea of taking a nap during the daytime?
4. Is there any one of your roommates who is not getting enough sleep? What is (are) depriving his/her sleep hours?
5. What suggestions can you give to your roommate concerning healthy sleep habits?

Section D   Follow-up Reading

Task 10   Reading Comprehension

Read the passage and fill in each blank with a proper phrase or sentence given in the box.

A study out today from the Centers for Disease Control shows a big chunk of the American work force, 41 million people get far too little sleep, and that's dangerous in more ways than one.

It's a nightly struggle waged by tens of millions of American workers —   1 , but many of us are losing. And today, the government put a number on it.

Unfortunately, what we found is that about a third of working adults get only six or fewer hours every day of sleep. Those most sleep-deprived are   2 , among health care workers, just over half said they don't sleep enough; for those in the transportation and delivery business, it was 70%.

Many studies have shown   3 , including heart disease, obesity and diabetes, and it is responsible for 20% of car crashes.

The CDC says people who work nights __4__. On the night shift at Brigham Young Hospital in Boston, some people like nurse Stephen Magarve say they actually do better working nights.

"Even when I was younger, I was a night person. I would have trouble sleeping at night, I was up all night", Magarve said.

But most like nurse Paula Ashy said they never catch up.

"I get on average maybe four hours a day, and even on my nights off, on average maybe three and a half, four hours sleep. Yeah, so I'm always tired," said Ashy.

A battle __5__ with no relief in sight.

_____	1.	A. they never catch up
_____	2.	B. those on the night shift
_____	3.	C. should adopt a regular sleep routine
_____	4.	D. would have trouble sleeping at night
_____	5.	E. with continuous exhaustion waged by millions
		F. beating the clock and somehow getting enough sleep
		G. a lack of sleep increases the risk for all sorts of health problems

Physical Exercise

Overview

Physical exercise is any bodily activity that enhances or maintains physical fitness and overall health. It is performed for many different reasons. These include strengthening muscles and the cardiovascular system, honing（磨练）athletic skills, weight loss or maintenance and for enjoyment.

Physical exercise is important for maintaining physical fitness and can contribute positively to maintaining a healthy weight, building and maintaining healthy bone density, muscle strength, and joint mobility, promoting physiological well-being, reducing surgical risks, and strengthening the immune system.

Frequent and regular aerobic exercise has been shown to help prevent or treat serious and life-threatening chronic conditions such as high blood pressure, obesity, heart disease, type 2 diabetes, insomnia, and depression. Strength training appears to have continuous energy-burning effects that persist for about 24 hours after the training, though they do not offer the same cardiovascular benefits as aerobic exercises do.

On the other hand, a lack of physical activity is one of the leading causes of preventable death worldwide. The World Health Organization（WHO）has defined physical inactivity as a global public health problem. Each year, approximately 3.2 million people die from causes related to physical inactivity.

Section A   Pre-audio-visual Tasks

Task 1   Glossary Work

Get familiar with the following words and expressions by listening to and reading them. Then complete each of the sentences with a proper word from the list.

intense /ɪnˈtens/ *adj.*	强烈的；紧张的
arthritis /ɑːˈθraɪtɪs/ *n.*	关节炎
depression /dɪˈpreʃn/ *n.*	沮丧；抑郁；萎靡不振
strengthen /ˈstreŋθn/ *v.*	加强；增强；巩固
release /rɪˈliːs/ *v.*	释放；公布
endorphin /enˈdɔːfɪn/ *n.*	内啡肽（体内产生有镇痛作用的激素）
debate /dɪˈbeɪt/ *n.*	争论；辩论；讨论
define /dɪˈfaɪn/ *v.*	界定；下定义
aerobic /eˈrəʊbɪk/ *adj.*	有氧的；需氧的
cardio /ˈkɑːrdɪəʊ/ *n.*	有氧运动
sit-up /ˈsɪtˌʌp/ *n.*	仰卧起坐
push-up /pʊʃ ʌp/ *n.*	俯卧撑
jogging /ˈdʒɒgɪŋ/ *n.*	慢跑锻炼
medium /ˈmiːdɪəm/ *adj.*	中等的；平均的
enhance /ɪnˈhæns/ *v.*	提高；增强
psychological /saɪkəˈlɒdʒɪkl/ *adj*	心理的；精神上的
statistically /stəˈtɪstɪklɪ/ *adv.*	统计上
evaluate /ɪˈvæljʊeɪt/ *v.*	评价；估价
compelling /kəmˈpelɪŋ/ *adj.*	令人信服的；非常强烈的
revealing /rɪˈviːlɪŋ/ *adj.*	揭露真相的；（服装）暴露的
aging /ˈeɪdʒɪŋ/ *n.*	老龄化；老化
strand /strænd/ *n.*	（线、纤维的）股；缕
consistent /kənˈsɪstənt/ *adj.*	一致的；连续的
suspect /səˈspekt/ *v.*	认为；怀疑（某事有可能属实或发生）
stress /stres/ *n.*	压力
build up	增进；建立
be attached to	附属于；喜爱

lifting weight	举重
work out	锻炼；解决；进展顺利
regardless of	不管；不顾

1. Call the doctor immediately if you _____ you've been infected.

2. A joke can be very _____ about what someone is really thinking.

3. He would need a very _____ reason to leave his job.

4. After many years of _____ study, he received his medical degree.

5. These exercises will _____ your stomach muscles.

6. They regularly walked, danced, ran and _____ at the gym.

7. During exercise, the body _____ chemicals in the brain that make you feel better.

8. People under a lot of _____ may experience headaches, minor pains and sleeping difficulties.

9. They are concerned with the physical and _____ well-being of their employees.

10. It's impossible to _____ these results without knowing more about the research methods employed.

11. She believes that success should be _____ in terms of health and happiness.

12. Many people suffer from clinical _____ for years before being diagnosed.

13. Over the year we have had several _____ about future economic policies.

14. You can _____ the flavor of the dish by using fresh herbs.

15. _____ is either acute or chronic inflammation of a joint, often accompanied by pain and structural changes.

Section B   Audio-visual Tasks

Task 2   Spot Dictation

Listen to a passage twice and while listening, you are to put the missing words in each numbered blank according to what you hear.

Intense physical exercise is not the only way to better health. Studies show that walking several times a week can lower the risk of many diseases. They include heart disease, stroke, diabetes, (1) _____ , arthritis and depression. Walking also can help you lose weight.

Fast walking is good for the heart. It lowers the blood pressure. It raises the amount of (2) _____ in the blood. Researchers say walking can sharply reduce the risk of suffering a heart attack.

Studies have also shown that walking for thirty minutes a day (3) _____ _____ and possibly prevent the development of type 2 diabetes. People who are overweight have an (4) _____ risk to develop this disease.

Walking strengthens the muscles and builds up the bones that they (5) _____ _____ . Studies show that women who walked and took calcium decreased their risk of (6) _____ , or thinning of the bones. Walking can also help ease the pain of arthritis in areas where bones are joined. This is because walking (7) _____ around the bones.

Walking several times a week is a good way to control weight and lose (8) _____ . Studies show it can also help ease the sad feelings of depression.

Experts say walking is one of (9) _____ to exercise. There is a low risk of injuries. So it is good for people who are starting an (10) _____ ____ for the first time and for older people.

Task 3　Short Answer Questions

Listen to the passage "Physical Exercise" twice. While listening, you are to give an answer as short as possible to each of the questions below.

1. What do endorphins released by the body do?

_____

2. What does the CDC define physical activity as?

_____

3. What are examples of muscle-strengthening activities?

_____

4. How much aerobic exercise should adults get each week according to experts?

_____

5. How much calories do people burn while running a kilometer?

_____

Task 4 Sentence Dictation

Listen to each sentence, repeat it aloud, listen to it again, and then write down the whole sentence in the space provided.

1. _____

_____

2. _____

_____

3. _____

_____

4. _____

_____

5. _____

_____

Task 5 Recognizing Details

Watch the video clip "Risks of Not Taking Exercise" twice and decide whether each of the statements below is TRUE (T) _or_ FALSE (F).

_____ 1. The new research of taking exercise was recently published in the _New England Journal of Medicine_.

_____ 2. The results of the study show that adults are doing well in taking exercise and have become more active.

_____ 3. The study results have proved that only about one third of adults can achieve the suggested physical exercise each week, which is 150 min. of light exercises.

_____ 4. It is revealed in the study that only about 15% of adults are sitting more than 6 hours a day, which shows that people have become more sedentary.

_____ 5. According to the research, lack of physical exercise will do harm to people's body and mind.

_____ 6. Working out is good to maintaining health and improving fitness both for children and adults.

_____ 7. Parents should set an example to their kids in taking exercise.

Task 6 Overall Comprehension

Watch the video clip "Exercise Linked to Longevity" twice and choose the best answer to each of the questions below.

1. Which of the following is mentioned as another compelling reason to stay physically fit?
   A. Doing physical exercise.   B. Cutting the risk of diabetes.
   C. Slowing the aging process.   D. Reducing the risk of cancer.
2. Researchers preferred to look at _____ for how old one's body is.
   A. blood sample   B. appearance
   C. longevity   D. individual cells
3. Cell aging is linked to _____ .
   A. how our bodies are aging   B. how quickly we get disease
   C. how intensely we get exercise   D. how quickly we get rid of disease
4. The critical marker researchers measured reflects that _____ .
   A. the shorter these strands, the older the cells
   B. the longer these strands, the older the cells
   C. the shorter these strands, the younger the cells
   D. the longer these strands, the shorter the cells live
5. What is a possible reason for people to have cells that look up to 10 years younger?
   A. Exercise helps reduce the stress that damages cells.
   B. Working out several times a week provides more energy.
   C. Exercising 30 minutes a day brings a good appearance.
   D. Exercise helps people overcome unpleasant surprises.

Section C Oral Tasks

Task 7 Listening & Interpretation

Listen to each sentence twice and interpret it into Chinese .

1. _____
   _____

2. _____
   _____

3. _____
   _____

4. _____
   _____

5. _____
   _____

Task 8 Dialogue & Conversation

Make dialogues and conversations , using the Chinese below as cues .

A：最近工作太多,搞得我压力山大。

B：也许你需要做些运动来振作精神。事实证明,定期体育锻炼有助于减少抑郁和焦虑症状来改善精神健康。

A：难怪经常锻炼的人总是活力满满,看起来也更年轻。

B：可现代人越来越不爱动、变得肥胖! 久坐的生活方式已成为一个全球性的公共健康问题。

A：看来每个人都应该热爱体育运动,养成有规律锻炼的习惯。

B：限制久坐时间和进行身体活动有助于促进减重,是健康生活方式的重要组成部分。

A：那我该做哪些运动来保持健康?

B：有不少运动方式可以保持健康。比如,世界卫生组织建议所有成年人每周至少进行 150～300 分钟的适度有氧运动。

A：什么是有氧运动？我可以做哪些有氧运动呢？

B：有氧运动是指人体在氧气充分供应的情况下进行的体育锻炼。有氧运动有游泳、步行、慢跑、滑冰、骑自行车、打太极拳、跳健身舞等。

Task 9 Discussion or Oral Presentation

Discuss briefly in a pair-group or make a 2-minute oral presentation based on the following questions.

1. How often do you take physical exercise? What kind of physical exercise do you prefer? And why?

2. State different kinds of physical exercises and their respective benefits.

3. What kind of physical exercise would you advise for middle-aged people?

4. Why do many elderly people take physical exercise early in the morning? Is early morning exercise better than exercise at later afternoon or in the evening?

5. What are the benefits of creating a society that will help people be active and make cities easier for people to walk and cycle?

Section D Follow-up Reading

Task 10 Reading Comprehension

Read the passage and complete each statement with a proper phrase or sentence given in the box.

How old is your body? Most people measure it in months and years, but some researchers preferred to look at something much more revealing: your individual cells. And what they found is people who exercise regularly actually have younger-looking cells.

"Looking into our cells is actually a window into how our bodies are aging. So our cell aging is linked to how quickly we get disease, and to how long we live," said Professor Elissa Epel of University of California, San Francisco.

The researchers took blood samples from 2,400 people and measured a critical marker for how cells are aging. The longer these strands, the younger the cells. The study found a consistent trend, regardless of whether people smoked or were overweight. The more they exercised, the younger their cells.

"This is the first study that's shown a factor that actually prevents or slows cell aging. So it's very exciting," Epel said.

In fact, people who spend an average of 30 minutes a day exercising had cells that looked up to 10 years younger than people who did not exercise. Researchers suspect that exercise helps reduce the inflammation and stress that damages our cells. Dan Kalika, who is 66, works out several times a week.

"It doesn't surprise me, because everybody I know who exercises, certainly has the appearance and the energy of somebody who is much younger," Kalika said.

Just one more reason to keep moving.

1. How old is our body can be measured not only by our age, _____.

2. The examination of the individual cells provides us with _____.

3. The length of the critical marker in blood samples _____.

4. Regardless of a person's history of smoking or overweight, more exercise _____ _____.

5. It's not surprising that those who do regular exercise _____.

> A. have younger appearance and are more energetic
>
> B. a window into how our bodies are aging
>
> C. but also by how younger-looking we are
>
> D. an approach to fight against disease
>
> E. decides whether our cells are aging
>
> F. will slow his or her aging process
>
> G. but also by our cells

Weight Control

Overview

Obesity is a medical condition in which excess body fat has accumulated to the extent that it may have an adverse effect on health, leading to reduced life expectancy and increased health problems. People are considered as obese when their body mass index (BMI), a measurement obtained by dividing a person's weight in kilograms by the square of the person's height in meters, exceeds $30 \, kg/m^2$.

Obesity is most commonly caused by a combination of excessive food energy intake, lack of physical activity, and genetic susceptibility, although a few cases are caused primarily by genes, endocrine (内分泌的) disorders, medications or psychiatric illness. Evidence to support the view that some obese people eat little yet gain weight due to a slow metabolism (新陈代谢) is limited; on average, obese people have a greater energy expenditure than their thin counterparts due to the energy required to maintain an increased body mass.

Dieting and physical exercise are the mainstays of treatment for obesity. Diet quality can be improved by reducing the consumption of energy-dense foods such as those high in fat and sugars, and by increasing the intake of dietary fiber. Anti-obesity drugs may be taken to reduce appetite or inhibit fat absorption together with a suitable diet. If diet, exercise and medication are not effective, a gastric balloon (胃气球) may assist with weight loss, or surgery may be performed to reduce stomach volume and/or bowel length, leading to earlier satiation and reduced ability to absorb nutrients from food.

Obesity is a leading preventable cause of death worldwide, with increasing prevalence in adults and children, and authorities view it as one of the most serious public health problems of the 21st century. Obesity is stigmatized in much of the modern world, though it was widely perceived as a symbol of wealth and fertility (生育) at other times in history, and still is in some parts of the world.

Section A　Pre-audio-visual Tasks

Task 1　Glossary Work

Get familiar with the following words and expressions by listening to and reading them. Then match the meaning description or synonym with a proper word or expression in the glossary list.

intervention /ˌɪntəˈvenʃn/ *n.*	干预
moderate /ˈmɒdərət, ˈmɒdəreɪt/ *adj.*	适度的
nutritious /njuˈtrɪʃəs/ *adj.*	有营养的;滋养的
Atkins /ˈætkɪnz/ *n.*	阿特金斯(饮食法)
The Zone /ðəzəʊn/ *n.*	区域饮食法
Ornish /ˈɔːnɪʃ/ *n.*	欧尼许(饮食法)
dieter /ˈdaɪətə(r)/ *n.*	(旨在减肥的)节食者
regain /rɪˈgeɪn/ *v.*	恢复;重回;复得
influential /ˌɪnfluˈenʃl/ *adj.*	有影响力的
alcoholism /ˈælkəhɒlɪzəm/ *n.*	酗酒
causal /ˈkɔːzl/ *adj.*	具有因果关系的
stunning /ˈstʌnɪŋ/ *adj.*	令人震惊的
staggering /ˈstægərɪŋ/ *adj.*	难以置信的
indulge /ɪnˈdʌldʒ/ *v.*	沉溺;放纵
voracious /vəˈreɪʃəs/ *adj.*	贪吃的;贪婪的
stigma /ˈstɪgmə/ *n.*	污名
skinny /ˈskɪnɪ/ *adj.*	极瘦的
equation /ɪˈkweɪʒn/ *n.*	等式;平衡
insulin /ˈɪnsjəlɪn/ *n.*	胰岛素

perpetuate /pə'petʃʋeɪt/ *v.*	保持
comprehensive /ˌkɒmprɪ'hensɪv/ *adj.*	全面的;综合性的
contentious /kən'tenʃəs/ *adj.*	有争论的
nugget /'nʌgɪt/ *n.*	一条(信息);块状物
bulge /bʌldʒ/ *n.*	凸出部分
interval /'ɪntəvl/ *n.*	间隔;(数学)区间
fidget /'fɪdʒɪt/ *v.*	坐立不安;烦躁
lean /liːn/ *adj.*	瘦的
wiggle /'wɪgl/ *v.*	摆动;扭动
be tempted to	受诱惑做某事;极想做
magic bullet	灵丹妙药;妙招

1. not extreme; being within reasonable or average limits _____

2. inclined or showing an inclination to dispute or disagree, even to engage in law suits _____

3. to allow yourself or another person to have something enjoyable, especially more than is good for you _____

4. including all or everything; broad in scope _____

5. of or relating to or resembling skin; being too thin _____

6. to cause to continue or prevail _____

7. containing various ingredients which are good for health _____

8. the habit of excessive drinking; habitual intoxication _____

9. involving or constituting a cause _____

10. a mark of shame, discredit or disgrace associated with a particular circumstance, or person _____

11. having a lot of influence on someone or something _____

12. having a huge appetite; excessively eager _____

13. a medicine or other remedy with advanced or highly specific properties

   _____

14. a pause or break in activity; a space between two things; a gap _____

15. to make small movements, especially of the hands and feet, through nervousness or impatience

   _____

Section B Audio-visual Tasks

Task 2 Spot Dictation

Listen to a passage twice and while listening, you are to put the missing words in each numbered blank according to what you hear.

Doctors say obesity, also known as severe overweight, is a complex condition. A doctor may advise (1) _____ in addition to changes in behavior. But experts say the most successful weight-loss plans include a (2) __ _____ diet and exercise.

People who want to avoid (3) _____ have to balance the number of calories they eat with the number of calories they use. To lose weight, you can reduce the number of calories you (4) _____, or increase the number you use, or both.

Experts at the National Institutes of Health say to lose weight, a person should do an hour of (5) _____ physical activity most days of the week. This could include fast walking, sports or strength training.

You should also follow a (6) _____ and take in fewer calories than your body uses each day.

A recent study looked at four of the most popular dieting plans in the United States. Researchers at Stanford University in California studied more than 300 (7) _____, mostly in their 30s and 40s.

Each woman went on one of the four plans: Atkins, The Zone, Ornish or LEARN. The women attended diet classes and received (8) _____ about the food plans.

At the end of a year, the women on the Atkins diet had lost the most, more than four and one-half kilograms on average. They also did better on tests, including (9) _____ and blood pressure.

Researchers at the University of California, Los Angeles, medical school found that most dieters regained their lost weight within five years. And often they (10) _____ even more. But those who kept the weight off generally were the ones who exercised.

Task 3   Note-taking

Listen to the passage "Obesity and Social Ties" twice. While listening, you are to take notes according to the cues given below.

1. Evidence that researchers have offered about obesity:

   _____

2. An effective tool in dealing with socially influenced problems:

   _____

3. A person's chances of becoming severely overweight if a friend has become obese:

   _____

4. A person's risk of becoming obese in same-sex friendships:

   _____

5. What the study shows concerning a major part of people's health:

   _____

Task 4   Sentence Dictation

Listen to each sentence, repeat it aloud, listen to it again, and then write down the whole sentence in the space provided.

1. _____
   _____

2. _____
   _____

3. _____
   _____

4. _____
   _____

5. _____
   _____

Task 5   Recognizing Details

Watch the video clip "Obese Nation" twice and decide whether each of the statements below is TRUE (T) *or* FALSE (F).

_____ 1. By the year 2030, a staggering 34 percent of Americans will officially be obese.

_____ 2. America is no longer a nation that loves to eat as Americans acknowledge obesity as a growing problem.

_____ 3. Those 100 kilograms overweight are classified as severely obese.

_____ 4. Not holding the waist line means bigger medical problems and health care bills.

_____ 5. Ms. Saber Basuto is trying to lose weight to be skinny and look great.

_____ 6. Weight gain is more than an energy equation or taking in more calories than you use.

_____ 7. A sedentary and overweight nation has something to do in a toxic environment.

Task 6　Overall Comprehension

Watch the video clip "Weight-Loss Secrets" twice and choose the best answer to each of the questions below.

1. Who can lose more weight and keep it off longer?

    A. People who lose weight slowly.

    B. People who lose weight steadily.

    C. People who lose weight fast.

    D. People who lose weight less.

2. Which is NOT mentioned as the option of intervals?

    A. Running.　　　　　　　　　　B. Walking fast.

    C. Zumba.　　　　　　　　　　　D. Swimming.

3. What do fidgety people NOT like to do?

    A. Sit.　　　　　B. Squat.　　　　　C. Wiggle.　　　　　D. Dance.

4. How can people fight against obesity through food?

    A. Drink one glass of white wine.

    B. Drink three glasses of red wine.

    C. Have small amounts of cocoa.

   D. Eat cookies.

5. How many secrets are mentioned in the video clip?

   A. 3   B. 4   C. 5   D. 6

Section C   Oral Tasks

Task 7   Listening & Interpretation

Listen to each sentence twice and interpret it into Chinese.

1. _____

   _____

2. _____

   _____

3. _____

   _____

4. _____

   _____

5. _____

   _____

Task 8   Dialogue & Conversation

Make dialogues and conversations, using the Chinese below as cues.

A:你对很多人在减肥这个现象怎么看?

B:这说明体重超重或肥胖已经成为公众健康的重要问题。

A:什么原因使体重超重的人越来越多?

B:原因是多方面的,有生物学的,也有生活方式方面的。

A:什么样的生活方式与肥胖有关呢?

B:生活方式包括饮食习惯和身体活动。现在不少人吃得多,活动少,是肥胖的促成因素。

A:为什么你说肥胖已经成为公众健康的重要问题?

B：这是因为超重或肥胖的人发生糖尿病、高血压、心脏病、卒中和某些癌症的风险更大。

A：难怪很多人在减肥，这确实是个重大的健康问题。

B：肥胖还是一个社会问题。在一个关注形象的社会里，肥胖的人或多或少会感受到一些偏见，因而会产生一些心理问题。所以，适当地控制体重，对保持身心健康是有积极意义的。

Task 9　Discussion or Oral Presentation

Discuss briefly in a pair-group or make a 2-minute oral presentation based on the following questions.

1. What is the definition of obesity? Is obesity a disease?
2. What are the possible causes of obesity?
3. What health problems can obesity cause?
4. What can a person do to keep his/her weight within the normal range?
5. Who are more concerned with their weight, men or women? And why?

Section D　Follow-up Reading

Task 10　Reading Comprehension

Read the passage and complete each statement with a proper phrase or sentence given in the box.

America is a nation that loves to eat. Despite what we all acknowledge as a growing problem, we are still tempted to indulge. Our voracious appetite is such that now one third of Americans are obese.

Today a new study projects that number will jump to 42 percent of adults by 2030. And those 100 pounds overweight, classified as severely obese, will increase by 11 percent.

A bigger nation means bigger medical problems and health care bills. But if we can hold the line, or more accurately our waist line, and not get any more obese, we could save $550 billion by 2030. We get plenty of encouragement from NFL football heroes to the first lady. For kids, weight carries more than just stigma.

"Older overweight children are more likely to have high blood pressure, to have higher cholesterol and to be able to move less well and play less well," said Dr. Eliana Perrin of University of North Carolina.

Saber Basruto lives with one of the consequences of childhood obesity, type 2 diabetes. She's lost weight, is on medication, and wants kids to learn from her. "It's not about being skinny or looking great. It's about being fit. Just eat healthier," Ms. Saber Basuto said.

But is weight gain just an energy equation, taking in more calories than you use? Or is it what we eat, refined sugars and grains that drive up insulin levels and can actually increase your appetite? One expert says it's not that simple. "We have a country that is perpetuating obesity because obese mothers are having children who are more likely to be obese as adults, and we have a toxic environment," said Dr. Janey Pratt of Massachusetts General Hospital.

And Dr. Pratt says that toxic environment consists of portions that are too big and Americans who constantly eat. So what does a sedentary and overweight nation to do?

Tomorrow we will get recommendations from the Institute of Medicine touted as comprehensive and evidence based, solutions that are likely to be as contentious at the many theories about the cause of our obesity problem.

1. One reason that one third of Americans are obese is they _____ .
2. One consequence that obese American suffer is they _____ .
3. For overweight children, they are more likely to _____ .
4. Saber Basruto wants kids to learn that losing weight is about _____ .
5. Experts believe that weight gain is a complex problem that _____ .

> A. have increase 42 percent
>
> B. have a voracious appetite
>
> C. have bigger medical problems
>
> D. being sedentary and overweight
>
> E. being fit rather than looking skinny
>
> F. have high blood pressure and higher cholesterol
>
> G. has to do with a toxic environment that people have

Eye on Women's Health

Overview

Despite obvious differences between women and men — biologically, psychologically, and socially — the concept of viewing the totality of women's health as different from men's health arose in Western medicine only in the last two decades of the 20th century.

Traditionally, the health of women has been seen as synonymous (同义的) with maternal or reproductive health. The modern field of women's health includes the study of illnesses and conditions that are unique to women, more common or serious in women, have distinct causes or manifestations (表现) in women, or have different outcomes or treatments in women. Since the 1980s, research on gender differences in health and disease has had important implications for the treatment and prevention of a variety of common serious illnesses, including heart disease, stroke, lung cancer, depression, colon cancer, and dementia (痴呆). Research in all these areas is ongoing.

The field of women's health seeks to promote an understanding of the biological and psychosocial factor affecting women's health, and to integrate this understanding into public health initiatives, including training of health care providers. Recognition by the medical research establishment of the need to study health and disease in women as well as men has been essential to this new paradigm (样式, 模式). Despite the strong influence of biological factors, psychosocial issues still remain the single most important determinant of health status for many women.

Section A   Pre-audio-visual Tasks

Task 1   Glossary Work

Get familiar with the following words and expressions by listening to and reading them. Then complete each of the sentences with a proper word from the list.

initiative /ɪ'nɪʃətɪv/ *n.*	主动性;积极性;倡议	
mammogram /'mæməgræm/ *n.*	乳腺 X 线片	
abnormal /æb'nɔːml/ *adj.*	异常的,不正常的	
guarantee /ɡærən'tiː/ *v.*	保证;担保	
invade /ɪn'veɪd/ *v.*	侵袭;侵入	
overwhelming /əʊvər'welmɪŋ/ *adj.*	压倒性的;势不可挡的	
anxiety /æŋ'zaɪətɪ/ *n.*	焦虑	
eventually /ɪ'ventʃuəlɪ/ *adv.*	最后;终于	
approach /ə'prəʊtʃ/ *v.*	接近;着手处理	
abdominal /æb'dɒmɪnl/ *adj.*	腹部的	
pelvic /'pelvɪk/ *adj.*	骨盆的	
urination /jʊərɪ'neɪʃn/ *n.*	排尿	
nightmare /'naɪtmeə/ *n.*	噩梦;梦魇	
pierce /pɪəs/ *v.*	刺入;刺穿	
indigestion /ɪndɪ'dʒestʃən/ *n.*	消化不良	
dismal /'dɪzməl/ *adj.*	凄凉的;悲惨的	
disconcerting /dɪskən'sɜːtɪŋ/ *adj.*	令人不安的	
unsatisfactory /ʌnˌsætɪs'fæktərɪ/ *adj.*	令人不满意的	
outright /'aʊtraɪt/ *adj.*	完全的;彻底的	
screening /'skrɪnɪŋ/ *n.*	筛查	
cervical /'sɜːvɪkl/ *adj.*	子宫颈的	
recession /rɪ'seʃn/ *n.*	衰退;不景气	
hormone therapy	激素疗法	
shrug off	不予理会;不予理睬	
a big deal	重要的事情	
on the go	忙忙碌碌的;不停奔走的	

red flag	危险信号
put sth. on the back burner	把……搁置
Pap smears	巴氏涂片检查
a silver lining	一线希望;好的一面

1. Experts stress the importance of _____ test for breast cancer for each woman each year.

2. Their social, moral and spiritual development is _____ .

3. The skills they need include creativity and _____ , the ability to make decisions and solve problems.

4. Fat which is built in the _____ region makes weight loss difficult.

5. High blood pressure may lead to complications, and _____ cause death.

6. People with urinary tract infections may feel a frequent urge to urinate and a painful, burning feeling in the area of the bladder or urethra during _____ .

7. They demand the _____ and immediate abolition of the tax on children's clothes.

8. Pap smears are effective tests to diagnose _____ cancer.

9. Physical exercise and low-fat-diet do not _____ a good health, because sometimes genes also play a role in determining a good health.

10. Diabetes is a chronic condition associated with _____ high levels of sugar in the blood.

11. Bacteria _____ human bodies and cause infection and inflammation.

12. A _____ usually refers to a bad and terrible dream.

13. Heartburn and _____ are usually caused by acid imbalances, and once we have them, it's very difficult to enjoy food.

14. Though the prospect of business is rather _____ , we should not be too worried about it.

15. An _____ majority voted to abolish abortion.

Section B　Audio-visual Tasks

Task 2　Spot Dictation

Listen to a passage twice and while listening, you are to put the missing words in each numbered blank according to what you hear.

　　Results from the Women's Health Initiative, a huge project in the United States, seem to have (1) _____ than answers. Many doctors are now wondering what advice to give their patients, especially older women. And many patients are wondering what (2) _____ to improve their health.

　　One of the major parts of the Women's Health Initiative was a (3) _____ _____. This involved studies of diet, hormone therapy and treatment with calcium and vitamin D. In the end, doctors did not find much of what they had expected to find. For example, doctors (4) _____ people for years to eat a low-fat diet. Studies have suggested that a diet low in fats and high in fruits, (5) _____ _____ might lower the risk of heart disease. Yet the Women's Health Initiative found no such link.

　　The women who changed their diet had a 9 percent lower rate of (6) _____ _____ than those who followed their usual diet. The reduction is considered small enough that it could have (7) _____ chance.

　　Yet the scientists say there are reasons to think it might not be the result of chance alone. For example, women who (8) _____ a higher level of fat in their diet, and did more to lower it, had greater reductions in breast cancer risk.

　　The findings from the tests of (9) _____ and vitamin D in the diet also surprised many people. The study found that these supplements offered only (10) _____. And there was no effect on the risk of colorectal cancer.

Task 3　Short Answer Questions

Listen to the passage "Controversy over Mammograms" twice. While listening, you are to give an answer as short as possible to each of the questions below.

1. What do many doctors think mammograms can do?

_____

2. What can the X-ray picture of mammograms show?

_____

3. What, according to some experts, does early discovery of breast cancer not always guarantee?

_____

4. What do some experts say long-term survival depends on?

_____

5. What will the National Cancer Institute continue to advise women in their forties and older to do?

_____

Task 4　Sentence Dictation

Listen to each sentence, repeat it aloud, listen to it again, and then write down the whole sentence in the space provided.

1. _____

_____

2. _____

_____

3. _____

_____

4. _____

_____

5. _____

_____

Task 5　Recognizing Details

Watch the video clip "High Alert Medical Symptoms for Women" twice and decide whether each of the statements below is TRUE (T) _or_ FALSE (F).

_____ 1. The news report is mainly about the warning signs of obesity and heart disease.

_____ 2. Barmer was diagnosed with thyroid disease, which is less common in women.

_____ 3. Women's health is more than reproductive medicine.

_____ 4. Consistent abnormal bloating pain could be a symptom of ovarian cancer.

_____ 5. Weight loss, frequent urination, constant thirst could be signs of early hepatitis.

_____ 6. Breast cancer is No. 1 killer of women.

_____ 7. Making about 70 percent of medical decisions in the family, women attach much importance to their own health.

Task 6　Overall Comprehension

Watch the video clip "The State of Women's Health in America" twice and choose the best answer to each of the questions below.

1. According to the report, the state of women's health in America today is _____.

   A. promising　　　　　　　　B. satisfying

   C. worrying　　　　　　　　D. prosperous

2. Which of the following is not mentioned as evidence of the state of women's health in America today?

   A. More women are too heavy.

   B. More women have high blood pressure.

   C. More women throw back too much alcohol.

   D. More women are under too much mental pressure.

3. According to Ms. Judy Waxman, who should be blamed for the falling health of American women?

   A. The local governments.　　　B. The World Health Organization.

   C. The federal government.　　　D. The Centers for Disease Control.

4. The highest percentage of diabetes in America is found in _____.

   A. Mississippi　　　　　　　B. West Virginia

   C. Texas　　　　　　　　　D. Oregon

5. All of the following are reasons why the report card is so dismal EXCEPT

   _____.

A. women usually ignore their own health

B. there are insurance issues in some states

C. there is a lack of access to good care

D. more women are dying from heart disease

Section C Oral Tasks

Task 7 Listening & Interpretation

Listen to each sentence twice and interpret it into Chinese.

1. _____

   _____

2. _____

   _____

3. _____

   _____

4. _____

   _____

5. _____

   _____

Task 8 Dialogue & Conversation

Make dialogues and conversations, using the Chinese below as cues.

A:通常一提到女性健康,人们往往就会想到孕产妇健康或者生殖健康。但其实远非如此。

B:那女性健康到底包括什么呢?

A:现代意义上的女性健康包括研究女性特有的、常见或严重的、在女性身上有不同原因或表现、或对女性有不同结果或治疗方法的疾病。

B:在日常生活中,女性容易患哪些疾病呢?

A:女性的常见病有很多,如甲状腺疾病、乳腺疾病、生殖系统疾病等,而女性健康的头号隐形杀手是心脏病。

B:看来女性迫切需要了解这些疾病的风险因素,从而有效地加以预防。

A:但是从社会心理的角度来说,女性作为照料者的角色使得她们常常忽略自身的健康。

B:是啊! 女性确实承受着巨大的角色冲突的压力,给她们的身心健康带来了巨大挑战。

A:一个家庭中70%的医疗决定都是女性作出的。女性健康关系重大啊!

B:确实如此! 关注与促进女性健康和福祉将造福全社会!

Task 9 Discussion or Oral Presentation

Discuss briefly in a pair-group or make a 2-minute oral presentation based on the following questions.

1. Why particular attention needs to be paid to risk factors for women's health?

2. What high alert signs and symptoms for women should never be shrugged off?

3. Give one or two examples to illustrate different clinical manifestations of the same illness in men and women.

4. What do you think of the government's role in promoting women's health?

5. What do you think women should do to properly manage their health?

Section D Follow-up Reading

Task 10 Reading Comprehension

Read the passage and complete each statement with a proper phrase or sentence given in the box.

There is a new report about the state of women's health in America. It is dismal, in a word. More women than just a few years ago are too heavy, have bad blood pressure numbers that are too high, and are throwing back too much alcohol.

In a 10-year look at women's health in this country, the National Women's Law Center reports that when it comes to meeting government goals to keep women healthy, the United States is failing.

"It's disconcerting that we have seen so little change over the last 10 years and

I think we really need to pay more attention and do more in the coming decade," said Ms. Michelle Berlin of Oregon Health Sciences University.

While no state is given an overall satisfactory grade, 37 states are found to be unsatisfactory, 12 considered outright failures, getting a grade of F.

"What the worst states did so wrong was not put into place policies that could actually help women get healthier. They did not do campaigns, education campaigns, to help women know what they could do to get healthier," said Ms. Judy Waxman of National Women's Law Center.

There has been some progress reducing deaths from heart disease, stroke, breast and lung cancer, but more women are obese and suffer from high blood pressure and diabetes.

"Certain states make an effort to help their women become healthier and it shows," Ms. Waxman said.

More than 33 percent of women in Mississippi are obese, the highest rate in the nation. And 13 percent of women in West Virginia have diabetes, also the nation's highest percentage.

Experts are concerned by the marked increase in the number of women who report binge drinking, and fewer women are getting Pap smears, the screening test for cervical cancer.

But there is some good news. Fewer women are dying from heart disease, stroke, lung and breast cancer. More women are getting mammograms, being screened for colorectal cancer, and even visiting the dentist more frequently.

There are a lot of reasons why this report card is so dismal. First of all, women take care of everyone else and put themselves on the back burner. There is a lack of access to good care in some parts of the country, insurance issues, and now of course the recession. But among the bad news, a little bit of a silver lining: women seem to be smoking less.

1. A 10-year look at women's health in the country showed that the United States _____ .

2. It's disconcerting that 37 states are found to be unsatisfactory and 12 considered outright failures, with no state _____ .

3. What the worst states did so wrong was not _____ that could actually help

women get healthier.

4. Some good news is that fewer women are _____ and breast cancer.

5. Women take care of everyone else and _____ .

A. put into place policies

B. failed to meet government goals

C. when it comes to women's health

D. given an overall satisfactory grade

E. put themselves on the back burner

F. dying from heart disease, stroke, lung

G. by the marked increase in the number of women

Promoting Teen Health

Overview

Although people change throughout their lives, developmental changes are especially dramatic in childhood. During this period, a dependent, vulnerable (易受伤的) newborn grows into a capable young person who has mastered language, is self-aware, can think and reason with sophistication, has a distinctive personality, and socializes effortlessly with others. Many abilities and characteristics developed in childhood last a lifetime.

A variety of factors influence child development. Heredity (遗传性) guides every aspect of physical, cognitive, social, emotional, and personality development. Biological factors such as nutrition, medical care, and environmental hazards in the air and water affect the growth of the body and mind. Economic and political institutions, the media, and cultural values all guide how children live their lives. Most important of all, children contribute significantly to their own development. This occurs as they strive to understand their experiences, respond in individual ways to the people around them, and choose activities, friends, and interests. Thus, the factors that guide development arise from both outside and within the person.

The study of child development is important for several reasons. One reason is that it provides practical guidance for parents, teachers, child-care providers, and others who care for children. A second reason is that it enables society to support healthy growth. Third, it helps therapists and educators better assist children with special needs, such as those with emotional or learning difficulties. Finally, understanding child development contributes to self-understanding. We know ourselves better by recognizing the influences that have made us into the people we are today.

Section A　Pre-audio-visual Tasks

Task 1　Glossary Work

Get familiar with the following words and expressions by listening to and reading them. Then match the meaning description or synonym with a proper word or expression in the glossary list.

overly /ˈəʊvəlɪ/ *adv*.	过度地;极度地
involve /ɪnˈvɒlv/ *v*.	包含;涉及;(使)加入
imbalance /ɪmˈbæləns/ *n*.	不平衡;不安定;失调
morality /məˈrælətɪ/ *n*.	道德;道德准则;道德观
medicate /ˈmedɪkeɪt/ *v*.	用药医治
psychiatry /saɪˈkaɪətrɪ/ *n*.	精神病学;精神病治疗法
Finland /ˈfɪnlənd/ *n*.	芬兰
diagnose /ˌdaɪəgˈnəʊs/ *v*.	诊断;判断
cognitive /ˈkɒgnətɪv/ *adj*.	认知的;认识过程的
symptom /ˈsɪmptəm/ *n*.	症状;征兆
inattention /ˌɪnəˈtenʃən/ *n*.	不注意;漫不经心;心不在焉
autism /ˈɔːtɪzəm/ *n*.	孤独症,自闭症
spectrum /ˈspektrəm/ *n*.	光谱;波谱;范围
severity /sɪˈverətɪ/ *n*.	严重;严重性;严厉
repetitive /rɪˈpetətɪv/ *adj*.	重复的;反复的
identification /aɪˌdentɪfɪˈkeɪʃn/ *n*.	识别;身份证明;密切关联
respond /rɪˈspɒnd/ *v*.	回答;回应;作出反应
stuffed /stʌft/ *adj*.	塞满的;吃饱的
puberty /ˈpjuːbətɪ/ *n*.	青春期,发育期;开花期
onset /ˈɒnset/ *n*.	发病;开始;攻击
pregnancy /ˈpregnənsɪ/ *n*.	怀孕期,妊娠期
abuse /əˈbjuːs/ *v*.	滥用;虐待;辱骂

cellphone /ˈselfəʊn/ *n*.	手机
distract /dɪˈstrækt/ *v*.	分散（注意力）；使分心
scan /skæn/ *v*.	扫描；浏览；细看
multitasking /ˌmʌltɪˈtæskɪŋ/ *n*.	多（重）任务处理
plasticity /plæˈstɪsətɪ/ *n*.	可塑性；适应性；柔软性
adolescent /ˌædəˈlesnt/ *n*.	青少年
Attention Deficit Hyperactivity Disorder	注意缺陷多动障碍；多动症
at large	一般说来；一般的；普遍的

1. lack of proportion or relation between corresponding things _____

2. to have or include (something) as a necessary or integral part or result

   _____

3. excessively _____

4. principles concerning the distinction between right and wrong or good and bad behavior _____

5. to identify the nature of (an illness or other problem) by examination of the symptoms _____

6. the branch of medicine concerned with the study, diagnosis, and treatment of mental illness _____

7. to administer a drug to (someone) _____

8. relating to cognition _____

9. a physical or mental feature which is regarded as indicating a condition of disease, particularly such a feature that is apparent to the patient _____

10. to make excessive and habitual use of (alcohol or drugs, especially illegal ones) _____

11. containing or characterized by repetition, especially when unnecessary or tiresome _____

12. the period during which adolescents reach sexual maturity and become capable of reproduction _____

13. the condition or period of being pregnant _____

14. the fact or condition of being severe _____

15. to prevent (someone) from concentrating on something _____

Section B   Audio-visual Tasks

Task 2   Spot Dictation

Listen to a passage twice and while listening, *you are to put the missing words in each numbered blank according to what you hear*.

Our subject is Attention Deficit Disorder, ADD, and the related form ADHD, Attention Deficit Hyperactivity Disorder. These affect an estimated five to ten percent of children worldwide.

Children who (1) _____ and never seem to finish tasks or pay attention might be found to have ADD. If, in addition, they seem (2) _____ ____ and unable to control their behavior, a doctor might say it is ADHD.

Experts say the cause involves a (3) _____ in the brain. It can affect not only school, but also personal relationships and the ability to keep a job later in life. Many of those affected also have (4) _____ or suffer from depression.

Medicines can produce calmer, clearer thinking for periods of time. But the drugs can also have (5) _____ like weight loss and sleep problems. And there is debate about the morality of medicating children.

Susan Smalley is a (6) _____ at the University of California, Los Angeles. She just led a study of ADHD in northern Finland. Prof. Smalley says medication is very effective in the (7) _____ . But she says the study raises important questions about the long-term effectiveness of (8) _____ __ .

The study also found that only about half the Finnish children diagnosed with ADHD had deficits in short-term memory and self-control. These (9) _____ ____ are generally considered part of the definition of ADHD.

The study also found more evidence that ADHD symptoms change with age. Hyperactivity and (10) _____ decrease. But about two-thirds of children continue to show high levels of inattention as teenagers.

Task 3   Note-taking

Listen to the passage "Early Intervention in Autism" twice. While listening, you are to take notes according to the cues given below.

1. Autism is a general term referring to:

   _____

2. Clear signs of autism are:

   _____

3. According to experts, another sign of autism may be:

   _____

4. Doctors and parents can also look for behaviors such as:

   _____

5. Examples of soft objects children like:

   _____

Task 4   Sentence Dictation

Listen to each sentence, repeat it aloud, listen to it again, and then write down the whole sentence in the space provided.

1. _____

   _____

2. _____

   _____

3. _____

   _____

4. _____

   _____

5. _____

   _____

Task 5   Recognizing Details

Watch the video clip "Early Puberty" twice and decide whether each of the statements below is TRUE (T) or FALSE (F).

_____ 1. More and more American girls are reaching puberty years before it used to begin.

_____ 2. Researchers have known why many American girls are growing up too fast.

_____ 3. Many parents are just scared about it because they have known this would cause other problems;

_____ 4. Dr. Joyce Lee is worried that girls who have earlier onset of puberty can be at higher risk for breast cancer and adult obesity.

_____ 5. The study conducted by Prof. Mary Wolff shows that the age of puberty is going down in the world at large.

_____ 6. Researchers believe the early puberty in girls is mainly due to poor diet.

_____ 7. Dr. Joyce Lee said chemicals found in everyday household products is another concern for the girls' earlier onset of puberty.

Task 6   Overall Comprehension

Watch the video clip "The Teen Brain and Electronics" twice and choose the best answer to each of the questions below.

1. What is the new major study about?

    A. How children are affected by the electronics devices.

    B. How the electronics affects the brain of all the children.

    C. How all of the electronics affects the brain of the average teenager.

    D. How parents are worried about the effects of electronics on their children.

2. Which of the following is a concern?

    A. Are our kids being taught to use electronics correctly?

    B. Are we teaching our kids to use electronic devices wrongly?

    C. Are our kids using electronic devices without being distracted?

    D. Are we raising kids who are constantly distracted by technology?

3. How long does the average child spend with media a day?

    A. 6 and a half hours.   B. 7 and a half hours.

    C. 9 and a half hours.   D. 11 and a half hours.

4. Dr. Jay Giedd scans the teens every two years to _____.

    A. test their distractibility

    B. understand their plasticity

    C. test their multitasking ability

    D. check their cross-training exercise

5. Which of the following statements is NOT true of Dr. Giedd?

    A. He's a parent of three teens.

    B. He wants to do the best for his children.

    C. He limits how much screen time his kids get.

    D. He also scans his teens' brain every two years.

Section C   Oral Tasks

Task 7   Listening & Interpretation

Listen to each sentence twice and interpret it into Chinese.

1. _____

   _____

2. _____

   _____

3. _____

   _____

4. _____

   _____

5. _____

   _____

Task 8   Dialogue & Conversation

Make dialogues and conversations, using the Chinese below as cues.

A:你认为影响青少年心理健康的因素有哪些?

B:现有研究发现有很多因素影响青少年心理健康:既有与同伴相处的压力,也有家庭生活和社会等因素。

A：你认为现在网络技术的普及对青少年心理健康有影响吗？

B：是的，我们无法忽视网络技术普及与青少年心理问题甚至青少年自杀之间的关系。

A：除了心理健康问题以外，青少年的其他健康问题是否也呈现上升的趋势？

B：最新的证据表明，儿童中的自闭症与多动症病例在增多。新近的研究发现，青少年的青春期提早了，尤其是女孩的青春期比以前早。

A：青少年的青春期提早是一种全球现象吗？

B：现在的研究无法证实这一现象，不过科学家们观察到美国的情况确实如此。

A：哪些因素影响到青春期早发？

B：这个问题只有在实证研究后才能得到解答。目前科学家们认为导致女孩子青春期早发的原因主要是青少年肥胖率的增加、饮食因素、缺乏运动和环境因素等。

Task 9   Discussion or Oral Presentation

Discuss briefly in a pair-group or make a 2-minute oral presentation based on the following questions .

1. Why is a growing attention paid to the children's health?

2. What important health problems concerning children's development need particular attention?

3. What is ADHD? What are symptoms and signs of ADHD?

4. Some parents are complaining that they are raising a generation that has never known a world without the internet or cellphone. What do you think those parents can parent better to help their children use electronic media smartly?

5. How, in your opinion, can the electronic media play a positive role in helping teens learn in this ever-changing world?

Section D   Follow-up Reading

Task 10   Reading Comprehension

Read the passage and fill in each blank with a proper phrase or sentence given in the box.

　　More and more American girls are growing up too fast, many reaching puberty years before it used to begin. And while researchers still aren't sure why this is happening or just how early puberty is taking hold, they ___1___.

　　Parents are worried about a new study from *Pediatrics* making headlines today. "We're just scared about it because we didn't know if this was something that was going to cause other problems years down the road," said Shonda Lewis, a concerned mother.

　　Shonda Lewis' anxiety seems to be supported by the study, which suggests that American girls ___2___. If true, concerning news. "Girls who have earlier onset of puberty are at risk, or at higher risk for earlier onset of sexual initiation and teenage pregnancy, as well as earlier onset of substance abuse, and in the long term these girls can be at risk for breast cancer and adult obesity," said Dr. Joyce Lee, a pediatric endocrinologist, University of Michigan.

　　But what does this study really say? "Now many of the headlines about this study ___3___. Is that a fair conclusion from the study?" asked Dr. Richard Besser.

　　"I don't think from this study we can say that the age is going down in the world at large," answered Prof. Mary Wolff, Preventive Medicine, Mount Sinai.

　　So despite all the press reports, the girls of this study are not representative of the general population. In some cases, they were selected because they ___4___. "This study was not actually designed to look at whether puberty was happening earlier or not," Prof. Mary Wolff explained.

　　But the trend is going in the wrong direction. With many other studies indicating that girls do face puberty earlier, researchers believe there are several key reasons: increased rates of obesity in children, poor diet, declining physical activity and chemical and environmental factors.

　　In fact, the authors of the study are actually in the first year of a long-term study, trying to ___5___. "We've done studies to show that heavier girls do have earlier onset of puberty, but the other issue of growing concern is chemicals that are found in everyday household products," said Dr. Joyce Lee.

　　Critical information for parents hoping to protect their daughters.

_____ 1.

_____ 2.

_____ 3.

_____ 4.

_____ 5.

A. were undergoing earlier puberty

B. are entering puberty earlier than ever

C. are concerned about the consequences

D. had existing risk factors for early puberty

E. had associated with chemical and environmental factors

F. were that the age of onset of puberty is going down dramatically

G. understand whether chemicals in the environment cause early puberty

Environment and Health

Overview

Environmental health is the branch of public health that is concerned with all aspects of the natural and built environment that may affect human health.

Environmental health addresses all human health-related aspects of both the natural environment and the built environment. Environmental health concerns include:

- Air quality, including both ambient （周围的） outdoor air and indoor air quality, which also comprises concerns about environmental tobacco smoke.
- Climate change and its effects on health.
- Disaster preparedness and response.
- Food safety, including in agriculture, transportation, food processing, wholesale and retail distribution and sale.
- Childhood lead poisoning prevention.
- Land use planning, including smart growth.
- Liquid waste disposal, including city waste water treatment plants and on-site waste water disposal systems, such as septic tank systems and chemical toilets.
- Medical waste management and disposal.
- Noise pollution control.
- Occupational health and industrial hygiene.
- Safe drinking water.

- Solid waste management，including landfills，recycling facilities，composting and solid waste transfer stations.
- Toxic chemical exposure whether in consumer products， housing， workplaces，air，water or soil.
- Vector（传病媒介）control，including the control of mosquitoes（蚊子）， rodents（啮齿动物），flies，cockroaches（蟑螂）and other animals that may transmit pathogens.

Section A Pre-audio-visual Tasks

Task 1 Glossary Work

Get familiar with the following words and expressions by listening to and reading them . Then complete each of the sentences with a proper word from the list .

particle /ˈpɑːtɪkl/ *n .*	微粒；粒子
pollutant /pəˈluːtənt/ *n .*	污染物
soot /sʊt/ *n .*	煤烟；烟灰
biodiversity /ˌbaɪəʊdaɪˈvɜːsətɪ/ *n .*	生物多样性
vulnerable /ˈvʌlnərəbl/ *adj .*	易患病的；易受伤的
ecosystem /ˈiːkəʊsɪstəm/ *n .*	生态系统
pathogen /ˈpæθədʒən/ *n .*	致病菌；病原体
esthetic /iːsˈθɛtɪk/ *adj .*	美学的；审美的
ethical /ˈeθɪkl/ *adj .*	伦理的；道德的
conservation /ˌkɒnsəˈveɪʃn/ *n .*	保存；保护
conversion /kənˈvɜːʃn/ *n .*	转换；转变
invasive /ɪnˈveɪsɪv/ *adj .*	侵害性的；蔓延性的；扩散性的
overharvesting /ˈəʊvə ˈhɑːvɪstɪŋ/ *n .*	过度获取；过捕
buffer /ˈbʌfə(r)/ *n .*	起缓冲作用的人（物）
allergy /ˈælədʒɪ/ *n .*	过敏；过敏性反应
photosynthesis /ˌfəʊtəʊˈsɪnθəsɪs/ *n .*	光合作用
formaldehyde /fɔːˈmældɪhaɪd/ *n .*	甲醛
benzene /ˈbenziːn/ *n .*	苯
volatile /ˈvɒlətaɪl/ *adj .*	易变的；不稳定的；易挥发的
pollen /ˈpɒlən/ *n .*	花粉

aggravate /ˈæɡrəveɪt/ v.	加重;使恶化
humidity /hjuːˈmɪdətɪ/ n.	湿度;潮湿
guilty /ˈɡɪltɪ/ adj.	内疚的;有罪的
synthetic /sɪnˈθetɪk/ adj.	合成的;人造的
ceramic /səˈræmɪk/ adj.	陶器的;陶瓷的
proactive /ˌprəʊˈæktɪv/ adj.	积极主动的;前摄的
sulfur dioxide /ˈsʌlfə daɪˈɒksaɪd/ n.	二氧化硫
nitrogen oxide /ˈnaɪtrədʒən ˈɒksaɪd/ n.	氧化氮
carbon dioxide /ˌkɑːbən daɪˈɒksaɪd/ n.	二氧化碳
carbon monoxide /ˌkɑːbən mɒˈnɒksaɪd/ n.	一氧化碳

1. Researchers are conducting a new National Biological Survey to protect species habitat and _____ .

2. Microorganisms, viruses, and toxins are examples of _____ .

3. They're afraid that we might _____ an already bad situation.

4. Now most people think that ecological awareness and environmental _____ depends on what we know scientifically about the natural world.

5. Companies are going to have to be more _____ about environmental management.

6. _____ is a gas that is produced when people and animals breathe out or when certain fuels are burned.

7. Carbon monoxide is a _____ that is formed as a product of the incomplete combustion of carbon or a carbon compound.

8. I don't mind hot weather, but I hate this high _____ .

9. He must have done something wrong, because he's looking so _____ .

10. Her skin problems are caused by an _____ to pollen.

11. Some doctors feel that this procedure is not medically _____ .

12. Like many actors, he had a rather _____ temper and can't have been easy to live with.

13. The virus leaves sufferers _____ to a range of infections.

14. They treated the cancer with minimally _____ surgery.

15. There is not a _____ of evidence to support their claim.

Section B   Audio-visual Tasks

Task 2   Spot Dictation

Listen to a passage twice and while listening, you are to put the missing words in each numbered blank according to what you hear.

Researchers have completed a major study on the (1) _____ of air pollution common in many large American cities. The study shows that air pollution increases the risk of death from lung cancer and other diseases.

The latest study (2) _____ in more than 100 American cities. The researchers examined their health records from (3) _____ . They also gathered information about air pollution in the cities where the people lived.

Researchers say the higher lung cancer risk (4) _____ pollution caused by small particles of soot from coal-burning power centers, factories and (5) __ _____ .

Power centers built before 1980 produce about half the nation's electricity. However, they also produce most of the power industry's (6) _____ . These include sulfur dioxide, nitrogen oxide and soot. Air pollution levels have decreased during the past 20 years because of (7) _____ of clean air laws. Yet levels of small particle pollution in major cities are at or (8) _____ _____ set by the Environmental Protection Agency.

Experts who have spent years examining the links between (9) _____ ____ generally support the latest study. The Environmental Protection Agency says it will consider the research as part of its continuing study of (10) _____ __ on small particle pollution.

Task 3   Short Answer Questions

Listen to the passage "Biodiversity and Human Health" twice. While listening, you are to give an answer as short as possible to each of the questions below.

1. What can animals, plants and microbes act as?

_____

2. What are examples of services that biodiversity is actually providing to us?

_____

3. What, according to Felicia Keesing, is the biggest threat that biodiversity faces?

_____

4. What, according to scientists, could a loss of biodiversity mean?

_____

5. Why is there no reason to delay protecting the Earth's ecosystems?

_____

Task 4　Sentence Dictation

Listen to each sentence, repeat it aloud, listen to it again, and then write down the whole sentence in the space provided.

1. _____

_____

2. _____

_____

3. _____

_____

4. _____

_____

5. _____

_____

Task 5　Recognizing Details

Watch the video clip "Super Plants Help Clean the Air" twice and decide whether each of the statements below is TRUE (T) _or_ FALSE (F).

_____ 1. Certain house plants might be able to fix more polluted air outside your home.

_____ 2. Bamboo is among better plants for improving air quality.

_____ 3. Photosynthesis is a process in which plants take in carbon dio-xide and put out oxygen.

_____ 4. Carbon monoxide, formaldehyde and benzene are stable organic com-pounds.

_____ 5. According to experts, more energy-efficient and air-tight apartments are more resistant to pollution.

_____ 6. Some of the better air-purifying plants may aggravate allergies.

_____ 7. Most of the super plants have no disadvantages in the house.

Task 6   Overall Comprehension

Watch the video clip "Environmental Cancer Risks" twice and choose the best answer to each of the questions below.

1. Which of the following has not been mentioned as a risk of getting cancer?

   A. Our genetics.   B. Household products.

   C. Polluted air.   D. Lifestyle choices.

2. Gail McDonnell is as guilty as anyone because _____.

   A. her children may be affected by cell phones

   B. cellphones have caused cancer in her children

   C. her children begin to worry environmental factors

   D. many Americans worry environmental factors

3. Environmental causes of cancer have been grossly underestimated because _____.

   A. more than 80,000 chemicals are used in the United States

   B. only a few hundred chemicals have been tested for safety

   C. Americans' fears of cancer have not been largely addressed

   D. most Americans have close to 200 synthetic chemicals in their body

4. All of the following are recommendations EXCEPT _____.

   A. filtering home tap water

   B. limiting the use of cellphones

   C. using ceramic or glass containers

   D. eliminating chemicals in daily products

5. The report's authors _____.

   A. are trying to scare people

   B. do not worry about anything

   C. try to evaluate environmental risks

   D. tell us not to worry about their point

Section C Oral Tasks

Task 7   Listening & Interpretation

Listen to each sentence twice and interpret it into Chinese.

1. _____

   _____

2. _____

   _____

3. _____

   _____

4. _____

   _____

5. _____

   _____

Task 8   Dialogue & Conversation

Make dialogues and conversations, using the Chinese below as cues.

A：人类生活环境在不断变化，人们对环境变化问题越来越关注。

B：引起人类生活环境变化有哪些因素呢?

A：人类本身的活动是生活环境变化的最重要影响因素，如人口增长、空气污染、固体垃圾及化学物处理等。此外，全球气候变暖、沙漠化、自然灾害等也是重要因素。

B：您提到的这些因素对公众健康与生活质量的影响如何?

A：大量研究表明，环境因素对公众健康有极大的影响。根据世界卫生组织估计每年大约有 1300 万人的死亡是由环境问题引起，而这些环境问题是可以预防的。

B：健康的环境对人们的生活质量与健康生活确实至关重要。影响公众健康的环境相关因素还有哪些?

A：其他因素包括辐射危害、病毒与细菌、饮用水安全、公共卫生服务基础设施薄弱等。

B：个人、机构与政府可以而且应当采取有效措施来保护环境。

A: 是的。我们需要个人和集体的公共卫生行动,必须清醒认识到,健康不仅仅是指个人的身心健康,还包括社会环境的健康。

B: 您说得对极了。一个健康的社会环境是公众健康生活的保障。

Task 9   Discussion or Oral Presentation

Discuss briefly in a pair-group or make a 2-minute oral presentation based on the following questions.

1. What are major environmental factors closely related to the public health?
2. What are major environmental problems in the region where you live?
3. What are sources of indoor pollution?
4. What is a healthy environment? Why is it important to our health?
5. What can and should be done to achieve a Beautiful China?

Section D   Follow-up Reading

Task 10   Reading Comprehension

Read the passage and complete each statement with a proper phrase or sentence given in the box.

The risk of getting cancer is often linked to our genetics and our choices like smoking, but today a presidential panel said it's time to take a hard look at the environment for potentially cancer-causing chemicals in our daily lives, like the water we drink and the household products we use.

Like many Americans, Gail McDonnell worries environmental factors like cell-phones may one day cause cancer in her children, reports CBS News medical correspondent Dr. Jon LaPook.

"They see — and I'm as guilty as anyone — all we moms on the phone, on the blackberry, and they start to mimic it," says McDonnell.

Today's report says more research should address fears like hers. The authors say environmental causes of cancer have been grossly underestimated. "We think environmental factors are causing cancer," says Dr. Lasalle Leffall of the President's cancer panel.

The presidential panel notes more than 80,000 chemicals are used in the

United States and only a few hundred have been tested for safety. "Most Americans all across the United States have close to 200 synthetic chemicals in their body," says Dr. Philip Landrigan of the Mount Sinai School of Medicine.

The report says so far there is no conclusive evidence that some chemicals found in everyday products cause cancer. However, it recommends certain lifestyle changes. For example, even with no proof cellphones cause brain cancer, the group advises limiting their use or wearing a headset.

Other recommendations include:

- Avoid microwaving with plastic containers; use ceramic or glass instead;
- Filter home tap water to remove possible toxins;
- Check home levels of Radon, a naturally occurring gas that causes an estimated 21,000 lung cancer deaths every year.

"Maybe the research at the end of the day will tell us there's nothing to worry about," says McDonnell. "But in the interim I want to be proactive."

The report's authors are not trying to scare people. Their point is that even though the impact of things like chemicals and cellphone waves are hard to evaluate, we've got to evaluate them.

1. The risk of getting cancer _____ and our choices, but today it's time to take a hard look at the environment.

2. Many Americans worry environmental factors like cellphones may _____ one day.

3. The authors of the report say environmental causes of cancer _____ .

4. The presidential panel notes only a few hundred of chemicals _____ .

5. The report recommends _____ using ceramic or glass instead.

> A. trying to scare people
> B. have been tested for safety
> C. cause cancer in the children
> D. is often linked to our genetics
> E. have been grossly underestimated
> F. recommends certain lifestyle changes
> G. avoiding microwaving with plastic containers

Stress Management

Overview

Stress, either physiological, biological, or psychological is an organism's response to a stressor such as an environmental condition. Stress is the body's method of reacting to a condition such as a threat, challenge or physical and psychological barrier.

Stress can alter memory functions, reward, immune function, metabolism and susceptibility to diseases. Disease risk is particularly pertinent (相关的) to mental illnesses, whereby chronic or severe stress remains a common risk factor for several mental illnesses.

When humans are under chronic stress, permanent changes in their physiological, emotional, and behavioral responses may occur. Chronic stress can include events such as caring for a spouse with dementia, or may result from brief focal events that have long term effects. Studies have also shown that psychological stress may directly contribute to the disproportionately (不相称地) high rates of coronary heart disease morbidity (发病率) and mortality.

Even though psychological stress is often connected with illness or disease, most healthy individuals can still remain disease-free after being confronted with chronic stressful events. This suggests that there are individual differences in vulnerability to the potential pathogenic effects of stress; individual differences in vulnerability arise due to both genetic and psychological factors. Research suggests chronic stress at a young age can have lifelong effects on the biological, psychological，and behavioral responses to stress later in life.

Section A　Pre-audio-visual Tasks

Task 1　Glossary Work

Get familiar with the following words and expressions by listening to and reading them．Then match the meaning description or synonym with a proper word or expression in the glossary list．

unavoidable /ˌʌnəˈvɔɪdəbl/ *adj.*	不可避免的
productive /prəˈdʌktɪv/ *adj.*	有生产能力的；多产的
stressful /ˈstresfl/ *adj.*	有压力的
uncontrollable /ˌʌnkənˈtrəʊləbl/ *adj.*	难以控制的
genetics /dʒəˈnetɪks/ *n.*	遗传学
chronic /ˈkrɑːnɪk/ *adj.*	慢性的；长期的
max /mæks/ *adj.*	最高的；最多的
psychologist /saɪˈkɒlədʒɪst/ *n.*	心理学家
ease /iːz/ *v.*	减轻；缓解
mobilize /ˈməʊbəlaɪz/ *v.*	动员；组织
motivate /ˈməʊtɪveɪt/ *v.*	驱使；激发……的兴趣
heighten /ˈhaɪtn/ *v.*	提高；加强
adrenalin /əˈdrenəlɪn/ *n.*	肾上腺素
trigger /ˈtrɪɡə(r)/ *v.*	引发；触发
delicate /ˈdelɪkət/ *adj.*	微妙的；精致的；脆弱的
overstress /ˌəʊvəˈstres/ *v.*	施加过多压力
buster /ˈbʌstə(r)/ *n.*	消除方法；遏制者
obligation /ˌɒblɪˈɡeɪʃn/ *n.*	义务；责任
annoyance /əˈnɔɪəns/ *n.*	恼怒；使人烦恼的事
cortisol /ˈkɔːtɪsɒl/ *n.*	皮质醇；氢化可的松
impairment /ɪmˈpeəmənt/ *n.*	损害；损伤
culprit /ˈkʌlprɪt/ *n.*	罪犯；肇事者
potent /ˈpəʊtnt/ *adj.*	有效的；强有力的
saliva /səˈlaɪvə/ *n.*	唾液，口水
straightforward /ˌstreɪtˈfɔːwəd/ *adj.*	简单明了的；坦率的

meditation /ˌmedɪˈteɪʃn/ *n.*	沉思；冥想
prescription /prɪˈskrɪpʃn/ *n.*	药方，处方
interfere with	妨碍；干扰
fight-or-flight response	战或逃反应
adrenal gland /əˈdriːnl ɡlænd/	肾上腺

1. to subject to too much physical or mental stress _____

2. to cause something to become higher or more intense _____

3. easily broken or damaged; fragile; susceptible to illness or adverse conditions

_____

4. the feeling or state of being annoyed; irritation; a thing that annoys someone; a nuisance _____

5. to make (something unpleasant or intense) less serious or severe _____

6. to cause somebody to become ready for service or action _____

7. an instruction written by a medical practitioner that authorizes a patient to be issued with a medicine or treatment _____

8. the state or fact of being impaired, especially in a specified faculty _____

9. the action or practice of meditating _____

10. (especially of a disease) lasting for a long time and continually recurring

_____

11. hormone produced by the adrenal glands that increases the heart rate and stimulates the nervous system, causing a feeling of excitement _____

12. making you feel worried and nervous; causing mental or emotional stress

_____

13. to set an action or a process in sudden motion; be the cause of sudden reaction

_____

14. study of the ways in which characteristics are passed from parents to their offspring _____

15. to cause somebody to act in a particular way; inspire _____

Section B Audio-visual Tasks

Task 2   Spot Dictation

Listen to a passage twice and while listening, you are to put the missing words in each numbered blank according to what you hear.

Stress affects everybody every day. It is your body's reaction to physical, chemical, emotional or (1) _____. Some stress is unavoidable and may even be good for us. Stress can keep our bodies and minds strong. It gives us the push we need to react to an urgent situation. Some people say it makes them more (2) _____ and gives them more energy.

Too much stress, however, can be harmful. It may make an existing health problem worse. Or it can lead to an illness if a person is (3) _____ the condition. For example, your body reacts to stressful situations by raising your blood pressure and making your heart work harder. This is (4) _____ if you already have heart or artery disease or high blood pressure. Stress is more likely to be harmful if you (5) _____ to deal with the problem or situation that causes the stress.

Anything you see as a problem can cause stress. It can be caused by everyday situations or by (6) _____. Stress results when something causes your body to act as if it were under attack. (7) _____ can be physical, such as injury or illness. Or they can be mental, such as problems with your family, job, (8) _____. Many visits to doctors are for conditions related to stress.

The tension of stress can interfere with sleep or cause (9) _____ or sadness. A person may become more forgetful or find it harder to concentrate. Losing one's (10) _____ is another sign of an unhealthy amount of stress.

Task 3   Note-taking

Listen to the passage "Personality and Stress" twice. While listening, you are to take notes according to the cues given below.

1. The concept of personality:

2. Characteristics of "Type A" personality:

3. Characteristics of "Type B" personality:

4. The reason for many women to be better able to deal with stress:

5. Reasons why many working women are under severe stress:

Task 4　Sentence Dictation

Listen to each sentence, repeat it aloud, listen to it again, and then write down the whole sentence in the space provided.

1. _____

2. _____

3. _____

4. _____

5. _____

Task 5　Recognizing Details

Watch the video clip "Benefits of Stress" twice and decide whether each of the statements below is TRUE (T) *or* FALSE (F).

_____ 1. Stress actually may do us some good if it is not too much.

_____ 2. The bills, relationship tension or even children can be sources of stress.

_____ 3. According to Dr. Romani Duvasla, stress is everywhere and is all bad to people's health.

_____ 4. The natural stress is our fight-or-flight response and it heightens our senses.

_____ 5. Stress may trigger the inflammation, which does no good to our body.

_____ 6. Headaches and higher blood pressure may be signs of overstress.

_____ 7. Exercise can be one of the best ways to change your overstressed state.

Task 6   Overall Comprehension

Watch the video clip "Stress Can Damage Women's Health" twice and choose the best answer to each of the questions below.

1. A new research shows _____ .

    A. how women manage to balance family, work and obligations

    B. few women are aware of their stressful situation

    C. how stress can ruin a woman's health

    D. a blood test could save people's life

2. Cortisol disorder increases a woman's risk for all of the following EXCEPT

    _____ .

    A. diabetes   B. gall bladder disease

    C. thinning of the bones   D. cognitive impairment

3. Which of the following is NOT true of the study?

    A. In times of stress adrenal glands release adrenalin and cortisol.

    B. Cortisol may course through our systems at all hours.

    C. High cortisol may become an internal enemy.

    D. Men are more likely to develop heart disease.

4. Large amounts of cortisol can result in _____ .

    A. high sugar   B. high level of estrogen

    C. dizziness   D. weight loss

5. Solutions to de-stress include all of the following EXCEPT _____ .

    A. regular exercise   B. slowdown

    C. meditation   D. balanced diet

Section C   Oral Tasks

Task 7   Listening & Interpretation

Listen to each sentence twice and interpret it into Chinese .

1. _____
   _____

2. _____
   _____

3. _____
   _____

4. _____
   _____

5. _____
   _____

Task 8   Dialogue & Conversation

Make dialogues and conversations , using the Chinese below as cues .

A:经常听说在工作和生活中压力很大。压力到底是什么?

B:在心理学上,压力指一种紧绷和压迫感,是我们人体对外界变化或影响的一种反应。

A:你是说压力并不是很可怕的事情?

B:是的。可以说工作和生活中压力无处不在,有些压力是不可避免的,甚至对我们有益的。

A:压力对我们有什么好处呢?

B:少量的压力可以帮助我们提高反应,帮助我们应对紧急事件,等等。

A:什么情况表明一个人的压力过大了呢?

B:压力过大的症状包括一种被压垮的感觉、焦虑感、紧张、食欲缺乏、抑郁、失眠、头痛、胃肠道问题等。

A：看来压力过大是有害健康的。那如何有效地去应对压力呢？

B：性别和性格不同在应对压力上会有差异。但一个人的健康精神状态很重要。健康的精神有助于人们更容易地去应对压力。

Task 9　Discussion or Oral Presentation

Discuss briefly in a pair-group or make a 2-minute oral presentation based on the following questions.

1. What is stress? What life events may cause stress?

2. Everyone feels stressed from time to time. Why in modern times may people feel more stressed out?

3. Long-term stress can cause both physical and mental harm. Discuss some common harmful effects of stress on your body, on your mood and on your behavior.

4. In what sense is stress good for us?

5. Some people cope with stress more effectively than others. What advice would you offer to your classmates, your colleagues or your patients to cope with stress?

Section D　Follow-up Reading

Task 10　Reading Comprehension

Read the passage and fill in each blank with a proper phrase or sentence given in the box.

The *Health Alert* is now about stress and women. A study just released by the Families & Work Institute confirms what a lot of women already knew. There is not enough time to ___1___ . And new research tonight shows how all that stress can ruin your health. And a simple test could save your life.

Emily Buchler thought life, that at warp speed, that clock never seems to stop, was just life. "Responding to emails, trying to meet these crazy deadlines so that I can then get home to ___2___ ", said Emily Buchler.

Stress, fatigue, and in addition, weight gain, especially belly fat, are more than just a modern annoyance. They can be life-threatening symptoms and a serious cortisol disorder. "It ___3___ , risk of heart disease, thinning of the bones, cognitive impairment and depression," said Dr. Sherita Hill Golden of Division of Endocrinology and Metabolism.

The culprit is cortisol. Like adrenalin, cortisol charges out of our adrenal glands in times of stress. But constant stress sends cortisol coursing through our systems at all hours. The potent hormone, suddenly an internal enemy, creating fat, ___4___ . One new study found that people with high cortisol are 58% more likely to develop heart disease. Another found women are more susceptible than men. "A few years ago, with a demanding career and kids I was like Emily. But a routine hormone check — as saliva test similar to the one she took — gave me a shock," said ABC's Claire Shipman.

And the solutions are straightforward but tough: enough sleep, regular exercise, everyday activities to de-stress, Yoga, meditation, an hour with a good book. I started working out like Laurie Fisher did, who was also motivated by the test. "Before that I felt guilty, trying to set time aside for me," said Laurie Fisher. But while you may not meet the test, ___5___ to do the obvious: slowdown.

_____ 1.	A. making too much sugar, and sending it to the wrong places
_____ 2.	B. causes the risk for cognitive impairment and depression
_____ 3.	C. think of the new research on cortisol as a prescription
_____ 4.	D. increases a woman's risk for developing diabetes
_____ 5.	E. balance family, home, work and obligations
	F. pick up my kids and take dinner on the table
	G. having negative effects on women's health

Coping with Depression

Overview

Depression is a state of low mood and aversion to activity. Classified medically as a mental and behavioral disorder, the experience of depression affects a person's thoughts, behavior, motivation, feelings, and sense of well-being. The core symptom of depression is said to be anhedonia (快感缺乏), which refers to loss of interest or a loss of feeling of pleasure in certain activities that usually bring joy to people. Depressed mood is a symptom of some mood disorders such as major depressive disorder or dysthymia (心情恶劣); it is a normal temporary reaction to life events, such as the loss of a loved one; and it is also a symptom of some physical diseases and a side effect of some drugs and medical treatments. It may feature sadness, difficulty in thinking and concentration, and a significant increase or decrease in appetite and time spent sleeping. People experiencing depression may have feelings of dejection, hopelessness, and suicidal thoughts.

Depression is the leading cause of disability worldwide. The World Health Organization (WHO) estimates that it affects more than 300 million people worldwide — the majority of them are women, young people, and the elderly.

Depression is a major mental-health cause of the disease burden. Its consequences further lead to a significant burden on public health, including a higher risk of dementia, premature mortality arising from physical disorders, and maternal depression impacts on child growth and development. Approximately 76% to 85% of depressed people in low- and middle-income countries do not receive treatment;

barriers to treatment include inaccurate assessment, lack of trained healthcare providers, social stigma, and lack of resources.

Section A   Pre-audio-visual Tasks

Task 1   Glossary Work

Get familiar with the following words and expressions by listening to and reading them. Then complete each of the sentences with a proper word from the list.

depressed /dɪˈprest/ *adj*.	抑郁的;沮丧的
recovery /rɪˈkʌvərɪ/ *n*.	(身体的)恢复;康复
parenting /ˈperəntɪŋ/ *n*.	养育子女
assistance /əˈsɪstəns/ *n*.	协助;帮助
resource /rɪˈsɔːs/ *n*.	资源;物力
populated /ˈpɒpjʊleɪtɪd/ *adj*.	人口众多的
psychiatrist /saɪˈkaɪətrɪst/ *n*.	精神病医生;精神病专家
moody /ˈmuːdɪ/ *adj*.	喜怒无常的
spell /spel/ *n*.	一阵;一段短暂时间
unprecedented /ʌnˈpresɪdentɪd/ *adj*.	前所未有的;空前的
grief-stricken /ˈɡriːf ˈstrɪkən/ *adj*.	极度忧伤的
spouse /spaʊs/ *n*.	配偶
checklist /ˈtʃeklɪst/ *n*.	清单
lethargic /ləˈθɑːdʒɪk/ *adj*.	昏睡的;没精打采的
divorced /dɪˈvɔːst/ *adj*.	离婚的
hardship /ˈhɑːdʃɪp/ *n*.	艰苦
suicidal /ˌsjuːˈsaɪdl/ *adj*.	自杀的
poll /pəʊl/ *v*.	对……进行民意调查
trauma /ˈtrɔːmə/ *n*.	创伤;外伤
misdiagnose /mɪsˈdaɪəɡnəʊz/ *v*.	误诊
counselor /ˈkaʊnsələ/ *n*.	顾问
grieve /ɡriːv/ *v*.	使伤心;使悲伤
prevalent /ˈprevələnt/ *adj*.	流行的;普遍的
antidepressant /ˌæntɪdɪˈpresnt/ *n*.	抗抑郁剂
Preventive Services Task Force	(美国)预防服务工作组

apt to	易于
seek treatment	就医
be susceptible to	易患……;易感的
take aback	使吃惊;使惊呆

1. The biological species on Earth is disappearing at a(n) _____ rate.

2. If someone is _____, they are often unfriendly because they feel angry or unhappy.

3. Researchers are carrying out a(n) _____ to find out what people think about depression.

4. A(n) _____ or school psychologist can help identify practical solutions that make it easier for the child and family to cope day by day.

5. The book confronts the harsh social and political _____ of the world today.

6. Osteoporosis is more _____ in women than in men.

7. She's been very _____ and upset about this whole situation.

8. People need time to _____ after the death of a family member.

9. Pete was so depressed after his girlfriend left him that I actually thought he was _____.

10. African Americans are more _____ get sickle-cell anemia.

11. In many cases, doctors _____ patients or give them the wrong treatment or not enough treatment.

12. A _____ is a doctor who treats people suffering from mental illness.

13. Two of the glands most extensively concerned with the response to _____ are the pituitary and adrenals.

14. In fact, a heavy meal or one loaded with carbohydrates can make you feel sluggish and _____.

15. The patient was discharged from hospital after his complete _____.

Section B   Audio-visual Tasks

Task 2   Spot Dictation

Listen to a passage twice and while listening, *you are to put the missing words in each numbered blank according to what you hear.*

The World Health Organization says more than 120 million people worldwide suffer from depression. But many people may not know it can start at a young age. In the United States, for example, (1) _____ estimate that about five percent of adolescents are depressed.

Depression is a medical condition that causes (2) _____ of sadness. Depression interferes with daily life.

Common signs of depression are lack of energy, (3) _____ in things you once enjoyed, difficulty thinking, problems sleeping or eating and thoughts of death. Depression also (4) _____ by physical problems such as headache, back pain, and stomach sickness.

Often, people suffering depression do not realize their feelings of sadness are due to a medical condition. They do not (5) _____ .

Medical experts say depression can affect anyone. There is no way to prevent it. However, the disease can be treated successfully. The sooner an affected person gets medical help, the better the chances of a quick and (6) _____ .

Depression is a common illness in the United States. It affects about 20 million adults. However, as many as (7) _____ do not seek medical treatment for depression.

The Preventive Services Task Force (8) _____ a study that says doctors should test all adult patients for depression during normal (9) _____ .

Medical experts say patients can be successfully treated for depression with medicines or by talking with a (10) _____ who treats medical disorders.

Task 3   Short Answer Questions

Listen to the passage "Dealing with Depression" twice. While listening, you are to give an answer as short as possible to each of the questions below.

1. How many Americans suffer major depression at some point in their lives?

   _____

2. Which groups of people have the highest rates of depression?

   _____

3. What aspects of lives can be affected by depression?

   _____

4. Why does depression often go untreated?

   _____

5. Why do many depressed people avoid treatment?

   _____

Task 4   Sentence Dictation

Listen to each sentence, repeat it aloud, listen to it again, and then write down the whole sentence in the space provided.

1. _____
   _____

2. _____
   _____

3. _____
   _____

4. _____
   _____

5. _____
   _____

Task 5   Recognizing Details

Watch the video clip "Women & Depression" twice and decide whether each of the statements below is TRUE (T) *or* FALSE (F).

_____ 1. New numbers show that about 10% of Americans are taking anti-depressants.

_____ 2. Middle-aged men are two and a half times as likely to be on antidepressants as women.

_____ 3. About half of the women aged between 40 and 59 are on antidepressants.

_____ 4. Maria Garay, a housewife with two children, is severely depressed.

_____ 5. Doctors are not sure why depression strikes women more often than men.

_____ 6. Women are less likely to seek medical treatment for depression than men.

_____ 7. There is clear scientific evidence showing that hormones and life pressures make women more susceptible to depression.

Task 6   Overall Comprehension

Watch the video clip "Are You Really Depressed?" twice and choose the best answer to each of the questions below.

1. How often do millions of Americans suffer from depression?

    A. Once in a while in their lives.

    B. At least once in their lives.

    C. Once a year in their lives.

    D. More than once a year.

2. Researchers were very surprised by their own findings because _____.

    A. a quarter of Americans who appear to be depressed might not be

    B. a quarter of Americans suffer from depression once a year

    C. Americans who are depressed are likely to be grief-stricken

    D. Americans who suffer from depression might be behaving normally

3. Which of the following questions is not included in the checklist to diagnose patients?

    A. "Do you have lack of interest?"

    B. "Do you have loss of appetite?"

    C. "Do you have suicidal thoughts?"

    D. "Do you have a family history?"

4. What did researchers find when they polled over thousands of checklists?

A. Most of the clinical diagnoses are incorrect.

B. Few of the patients are dealing with trauma.

C. A significant number of cases have been misdiagnosed.

D. The checklists are too complex to be used clinically.

5. Although the checklists are too broad, many doctors think that _____.

A. there are many patients who need help

B. there is no possibility of misdiagnosis

C. more patients are to be labeled clinically

D. the checklists need to be revised clinically

Section C Oral Tasks

Task 7 Listening & Interpretation

Listen to each sentence twice and interpret it into Chinese.

1. _____

_____

2. _____

_____

3. _____

_____

4. _____

_____

5. _____

_____

Task 8 Dialogue & Conversation

Make dialogues and conversations, using the Chinese below as cues.

A：受学业压力等一些因素的影响，社会各界对学生的心理健康问题越来越关注。

B：是的。国家卫健委已提出，高中及高等院校要将抑郁症筛查纳入学生健康体检内容。

A：抑郁症筛查要怎么进行？ 填写一张调查表就可以了吗？

B：心理健康问题的筛查远不止发放问卷让学生填写这么简单。

A：您能否再详细解释一下？

B：心理测评是高度专业的工作,且有相关伦理要求。

A：那么心理测评表的制作有哪些要求呢？

B：心理测评表的制作一定要科学、专业,符合受调查者的特点。

A：如果筛查分数高就是得了抑郁症吗？

B：不一定。测评只是一种辅助手段。目前,全世界对抑郁症的诊断主要是通过医生和患者面对面的交谈,而不是通过简单的问卷来确诊。

Task 9   Discussion or Oral Presentation

Discuss briefly in a pair-group or make a 2-minute oral presentation based on the following questions.

1. What two or three most interesting things have you learned from this unit?
2. What are the possible causes of depression?
3. Which age group of people is more likely to suffer from depression? Why?
4. Have you ever had the experience of feeling depressed? How do you deal with the situation?
5. Why is there a gender difference in the depression rate?

Section D   Follow-up Reading

Task 10   Reading Comprehension

Read the passage and complete each statement with a proper phrase or sentence given in the box.

It's widely estimated that more than 30 million Americans will suffer from depression at least once in their lives. And depression is a very real illness with very real consequences. But a major new study out today finds that one out of every four people told they have depression, could in fact be reacting normally to some of life's more troubling times.

Researchers were taken aback by their own findings, arguing a quarter of

Americans who appear to be depressed might not be. Instead, they could be sad or grief-stricken just as anyone else would be.

"It's normal to be sad after your spouse dies. We're arguing it's also normal to be sad after another terrible thing happens, like you lose your job or you get divorced," said one psychiatrist.

Right now those other hardships are not considered when evaluating a patient. Hundreds of thousands of medical professionals use the same checklist issued by the American Psychiatric Association to diagnose patients with clinical depression. They ask: "Are you depressed? Do you have a lack of interest, loss of appetite, little sleep? Are you lethargic? Do you have fatigue, guilt, lack of concentration or, suicidal thoughts? Five or more of the symptoms and you're clinically depressed."

Researchers polled over thousands of those checklists and they saved all the people who wouldn't be labeled depressed. A significant number of them were dealing with a kind of loss and trauma. It would make any of us sad.

"Is it a possibility that there are people out there who've been diagnosed incorrectly?" David Muir asked.

"Absolutely. Absolute possibility," the psychiatrist answered.

And if they are misdiagnosed, is their treatment wrong too? All questions Kathy Anderson asks every day. She's now a counselor after having lost a son. She reaches out to others who are grieving, who she believes are too quickly labeled clinically depressed.

"I think it's just such a prevalent term that it's almost expected that we'll be depressed," Kathy Anderson said.

Still many doctors say the checklist, though simple and too broad, helps more than it hurts, arguing whether patients are labeled clinically depressed or not, they still need help.

1. A major new study has found that _____ .

2. Researchers argued that sometimes people were not depressed; they were just

_____ .

3. It is possible that _____ .

4. According to Kathy Anderson, _____ .

5. Many doctors hold that _____ .

A. in low spirits after experiencing a difficult time in life

B. fewer people will suffer from depression in the future

C. people might be misdiagnosed as having depression

D. it will become more challenging to fight against depression

E. sometimes doctors make depression diagnosis too quickly

F. 25% of Americans who appear to be depressed might not be

G. the benefits of the depression checklist outweigh its shortcomings

First Aid

Overview

First aid is the first and immediate assistance given to any person suffering from either a minor or serious illness or injury, with care provided to preserve life, prevent the condition from worsening, or to promote recovery. It includes initial intervention in a serious condition prior to professional medical help being available, such as performing cardiopulmonary resuscitation (CPR) while waiting for an ambulance, as well as the complete treatment of minor conditions, such as applying a plaster to a cut.

The primary goal of first aid is to prevent death or serious injury from worsening. The key aims of first aid can be summarized with the acronym of 'the three Ps':

Preserve life: The overriding aim of all medical care which includes first aid, is to save lives and minimize the threat of death. First aid done correctly should help reduce the patient's level of pain and calm them down during the evaluation and treatment process.

Prevent further harm: Prevention of further harm includes addressing both external factors, such as moving a patient away from any cause of harm, and applying first aid techniques to prevent worsening of the condition, such as applying pressure to stop a bleed becoming dangerous.

Promote recovery: First aid also involves trying to start the recovery process from the illness or injury, and in some cases might involve completing a treatment, such as in the case of applying a plaster to a small wound.

It is important to note that first aid is not medical treatment and cannot be compared with what a trained medical professional provides. First aid involves making common sense decisions in the best interest of an injured person.

First aid is generally performed by someone with basic medical training. There are many situations that may require first aid, and many countries have legislation (法律,法规), regulation, or guidance, which specifies a minimum level of first aid provision in certain circumstances. This can include specific training or equipment to be available in the workplace, or mandatory (强制的) first aid training within schools.

Section A   Pre-audio-visual Tasks

Task 1   Glossary Work

Get familiar with the following words and expressions by listening to and reading them. Then match the meaning description or synonym with a proper word or expression in the glossary list.

emergency /ɪ'mɜːdʒənsi/ *n*.	紧急;急症;意外
choking /'tʃəʊkɪŋ/ *adj*.	窒息的;憋闷的
rib /rɪb/ *n*.	肋骨
expel /ɪk'spel/ *v*.	呼出空气;排出
cardiopulmonary /ˌkɑːdɪəʊ'pʌlmənərɪ/ *adj*.	心肺的
resuscitation /rɪˌsʌsɪ'teɪʃn/ *n*.	复苏
drown /draʊn/ *v*.	(使)淹死;淹没
rescue /'reskjuː/ *n*.	援救;营救
collapse /kə'læps/ *v*.	虚脱
surrounding /sə'raʊndɪŋ/ *n*.	周围环境
chest /tʃest/ *n*.	胸部
compression /kəm'preʃən/ *n*.	压迫;压缩
airway /'eəweɪ/ *n*.	(肺的)气道;通气道
administer /əd'mɪnɪstə(r)/ *v*.	给予;施行
mannequin /'mænɪkɪn/ *n*.	人体模型
resume /rɪ'zuːm/ *v*.	重新开始;重返

reluctant /rɪˈlʌktənt/ *adj.*		不情愿的；厌恶的
emphasize /ˈemfəsaɪz/ *v.*		强调；重视
category /ˈkætɪɡərɪ/ *n.*		种类；部属；类目
faint /feɪnt/ *v.*		昏晕；昏倒
uncomplicated /ʌnˈkɒmplɪkeɪtɪd/ *adj.*		简单的；不复杂的
irreversible /ˌɪrɪˈvɜːsəbl/ *adj.*		不可逆的
paralysis /pəˈræləsɪs/ *n.*		瘫痪；麻痹
electrocution /ɪˌlektrəˈkjuːʃn/ *n.*		电击；电死
asphyxiation /əsˌfɪksɪˈeɪʃn/ *n.*		窒息
first aid		急救
heart attack		心脏病发作
the Heimlich maneuver		海姆利克操作法
the spinal cord		脊髓
slump over		伏倒

1. a collection of things sharing a common attribute _____

2. killing by electric shock _____

3. to pass out from weakness, physical or emotional distress due to a loss of blood supply to the brain _____

4. lacking complexity _____

5. incapable of being reversed _____

6. killing by depriving of oxygen _____

7. loss of the ability to move a body part _____

8. the process or result of becoming smaller or pressed together _____

9. to fall down and become unconscious as a result of illness or injury _____

10. an act of saving or being saved from danger or difficulty _____

11. to force to leave or move out _____

12. any of the 12 pairs of curved arches of bone extending from the spine to or toward the sternum in humans (and similar bones in most vertebrates) _____

13. a condition caused by blocking the airways to the lungs (as with food or swelling of the larynx) _____

14. a sudden unforeseen crisis (usually involving danger) that requires immediate

action _____

15. an emergency procedure to help someone who is choking because food is lodged in the trachea

_____

Section B   Audio-visual Tasks

Task 2   Spot Dictation

Listen to a passage twice and while listening, you are to put the missing words in each numbered blank according to what you hear.

First aid is the kind of medical care given to a victim of an accident or (1) _____ _____ before trained medical help can arrive. First aid methods generally are easy to carry out and can be taught to people of all ages. Learning them is important. Knowing how to treat someone (2) _____ can mean the difference between life and death.

Many emergency (3) _____ are simple and easy to carry out. For example, several years ago, a 5-year-old boy in the American state of Massachusetts was playing with a young friend. Suddenly the friend stopped breathing. A piece of candy (4) _____ in her throat.

The boy remembered a television program where the same thing had happened. He also remembered what people on the television program did to help the person who had (5) _____.

The simple method used by the 5-year-old boy is called the Heimlich maneuver. It (6) _____ by an American doctor, Henry Heimlich. The Heimlich maneuver can be done in several different ways.

If a (7) _____ is sitting or standing, you should stand directly behind him. Put your arms around the victim's waist.

Make one of your hands (8) _____ of a ball, and place it over the top part of the stomach, (9) _____.

Next, put one hand over the other and push in and upward sharply. Repeat the method until the object (10) _____.

Task 3   Note-taking

Listen to the passage "Cardiopulmonary Resuscitation" twice. While listening, you are to take notes according to the cues given below.

1. Cardiopulmonary resuscitation is performed to increase:

_____

2. One method of helping the victim without rescue breathing is:

_____

3. The conditions indicating a person is unconscious:

_____

4. Chest compressions can be done to help:

_____

5. What to do first for a choking victim who is unconscious with no heartbeat:

_____

Task 4　Sentence Dictation

Listen to each sentence, repeat it aloud, listen to it again, and then write down the whole sentence in the space provided.

1. _____

_____

2. _____

_____

3. _____

_____

4. _____

_____

5. _____

_____

Task 5　Recognizing Details

Watch the video clip "New Rules for CPR" twice and decide whether each of the statements below is TRUE (T) *or* FALSE (F).

_____ 1. In an emergency, the most important thing to do is administer CPR.

_____ 2. Red Cross always concentrates on the mouth-to-mouth component.

_____ 3. In the first aid, the most important thing is saving lives.

_____ 4. The compressions are done in the middle of the chest at the frequency of normal heartbeat.

_____ 5. Today's studies say that the compressions alone are just as good as compressions with breaths in CPR.

_____ 6. If you are not trained in CPR, you should do chest-only compressions.

_____ 7. You should take a CPR class at your local Red Cross or Heart Association office to administer CPR.

Task 6   Overall Comprehension

Watch the video clip "Emergency Care for an Unconscious Person" twice and choose the best answer to each of the questions below.

1. When you find someone who is unconscious, it is important to _____.
   A. take immediate steps to help that person
   B. determine how much you can help that person
   C. call for a medical professional as quickly as possible
   D. make clear how you find that person who is unconscious

2. If you see a person become unconscious while walking, talking or laughing, that could be a case _____.
   A. relatively uncomplicated   B. occurring very frequently
   C. that doesn't require CPR   D. very complicated to deal with

3. When you come across somebody who is unconscious, you don't know any of the following EXCEPT _____.
   A. what happened to him
   B. what his medical state was
   C. whether he had any underlined conditions
   D. whether he lacked consciousness and responsiveness to people

4. When you come across somebody who is lying down, the biggest thing to worry about is _____.
   A. irreversible paralysis
   B. potential asphyxiation

C. a head injury or a neck injury

D. cessation of heartbeat and breathing

5. If you come across the person who is unconscious, you need to be more cautious because _____ .

A. performing CPR may cause potential harm

B. there are many causes of unconsciousness

C. basic life support is a part of emergency help

D. emergency help is really a first important step

Section C Oral Tasks

Task 7 Listening & Interpretation

Listen to each sentence twice and interpret it into Chinese.

1. _____

_____

2. _____

_____

3. _____

_____

4. _____

_____

5. _____

_____

Task 8 Dialogue & Conversation

Make dialogues and conversations, using the Chinese below as cues.

A:作为医科学生,你对急救了解多少?

B:这个学期,我们刚刚在急救技能方面接受了培训。

A:你是怎么理解急救的?

B:急救是指对疾病或受伤提供初步处理。它通常是由非专家、但经过训练的人员对病者或伤者实施的,直到病者或伤者得到权威的治疗。

A:急救的目标是什么？

B:急救的目标可以概括成 3 个要点：保护生命、防止进一步伤害和促进康复。

A:哪些状况是经常需要急救的？

B:有不少状况都需要急救，如心脏病发作、骨折、心脏骤停、脑卒中、中毒、癫痫发作、烧伤、溺水或窒息等。

A:进行急救需要哪些方法和技能呢？

B:急救通常是由一系列简单的技术构成，一个人可以经培训后用最少设备来实施。

Task 9   Discussion or Oral Presentation

Discuss briefly in a pair-group or make a 2-minute oral presentation based on the following questions.

1. Have you ever met a medical emergency? How did you deal with it?
2. What does first aid refer to?
3. What are the situations in which first aid is often needed?
3. What are the aims of first aid?
4. What other knowledge do you have about first aid?

Section D   Follow-up Reading

Task 10   Reading Comprehension

Read the passage and fill in each blank with a proper phrase or sentence given in the box.

What do I do if I find someone who is unconscious?

The most important thing to remember is：Did you see this person become unconscious or did you come across this person when he or she was unconscious? And that's very important because that ___1___ and the steps that you actually take to help that person.

Now let's talk about the first category. Did you see this person become unconscious? They were walking, talking, laughing and all of a sudden maybe they fainted or they were in a chair and they slumped over. In that case you know that they were okay before that, so that could be something that's relatively uncomplicated, in most cases. And you can put that person on the floor, and you can see if they are breathing and __2__ and call 911 if they don't regain consciousness within a few minutes.

In a situation where you come across somebody who is unconscious, that's a completely different ball game and the reason for that is you don't know what happened to him, you don't know if they __3__, you don't know what their medical state was, you don't know if they are injured and so forth and so on.

The biggest thing to worry about is a head injury or a neck injury. So you come across somebody who is lying down, don't move them, that's really important because if there is a head injury or neck injury you have the potential to injure the spinal cord which __4__ and you don't want to be any part of that.

So the first thing you do is to call for help as quickly as you can, and then you __5__ and possibly perform CPR and basic life support for that person before emergency help arrives.

There are many, many causes of unconsciousness, such as head injuries, electrocution, asphyxiation, certain poisons, but again the most important factor is: Did you see this person become unconscious? Were they normal, walking, talking, laughing before that? Or did you come across the person when they were unconscious? And you need to be more cautious if you came across the person when they were unconscious.

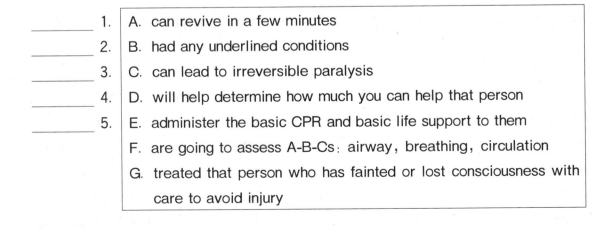

_____ 1.	A. can revive in a few minutes
_____ 2.	B. had any underlined conditions
_____ 3.	C. can lead to irreversible paralysis
_____ 4.	D. will help determine how much you can help that person
_____ 5.	E. administer the basic CPR and basic life support to them
	F. are going to assess A-B-Cs: airway, breathing, circulation
	G. treated that person who has fainted or lost consciousness with care to avoid injury

Preventing Epidemics

Overview

A pandemic is an epidemic of an infectious disease that has spread across a large region, for instance multiple continents or worldwide, affecting a substantial (重大的) number of individuals. Throughout human history, there have been a number of pandemics of diseases such as smallpox. The most fatal pandemic in recorded history was the Black Death [also known as The Plague (瘟疫)], which killed an estimated 75 - 200 million people in the 14th century. The term was not used back then but was used during later pandemics including the 1918 influenza pandemic (Spanish flu). Recent pandemics include Sixth Cholera Pandemic, Spanish Flu Pandemic, Asian Flu, Hong Kong Flu, HIV/AIDS, SARS, H1N1, and COVID-19.

A broad group of the non-pharmaceutical (非药物的) interventions may be taken to manage the outbreak. In a flu pandemic, these actions may include personal preventive measures such as hand hygiene, wearing face-masks, and self-quarantine (自我隔离); community measures which aim at social distancing such as closing schools and canceling mass gatherings; community engagement to encourage acceptance and participation in such interventions; and environmental measures such as cleaning of surfaces.

The basic strategies in the control of an outbreak are containment (控制) and mitigation (缓解,减轻). Containment may be undertaken in the early stages of the outbreak, including contact tracing and isolating infected individuals to stop the disease from spreading to the rest of the population, other public health interventions on infection control, and therapeutic countermeasures（对抗措施）such as vaccinations which may be effective if available. When it becomes apparent that it is no longer possible to contain the spread of the disease, management will then move on to the mitigation stage, in which measures are taken to slow the spread of the disease and mitigate（缓解，减轻）its effects on society and the healthcare system. In reality, containment and mitigation measures may be undertaken simultaneously.

Section A Pre-audio-visual Tasks

Task 1 Glossary Work

Get familiar with the following words and expressions by listening to and reading them. Then complete each of the sentences with a proper word from the list.

antibody /ˈæntɪbɒdɪ/ *n.*	抗体
pandemic /pænˈdemɪk/ *n.*	大流行病
barrier /ˈbærɪə(r)/ *n.*	屏障；障碍
infectious /ɪnˈfekʃəs/ *adj.*	传染的；有传染性的
glove /ɡlʌv/ *n.*	手套
candidate /ˈkændɪdət/ *n.*	候选人；适合……的人/物
defense /dɪˈfens/ *n.*	防御能力；防御；辩护
infect /ɪnˈfekt/ *v.*	传染；使感染
outbreak /ˈaʊtbreɪk/ *n.*	（战争、疾病等的）爆发；突然发生
transmission /trænzˈmɪʃn/ *n.*	传播；传送
propagate /ˈprɒpəɡeɪt/ *v.*	传播；宣传
positive /ˈpɒzətɪv/ *adj.*	阳性的；积极乐观的
strategy /ˈstrætədʒɪ/ *n.*	策略；部署
responder /rɪˈspɒndə/ *n.*	回应者；响应器
perspective /pəˈspektɪv/ *n.*	观点；看法
surgical /ˈsɜːdʒɪkl/ *adj.*	外科的；外科手术的
efficacy /ˈefɪkəsɪ/ *n.*	功效；效力；效验
fabric /ˈfæbrɪk/ *n.*	织物；结构

hygiene /ˈhaɪdʒiːn/ *n*.	卫生;卫生学
shield /ʃiːld/ *n*.	护罩;盾;保护人
avian flu	禽流感
COVID-19	新型冠状病毒病
contact tracing	接触者追踪
reach out to	联系;把手伸向
get out of control	失去控制
come up with	想出;想到
shed light on	为……提供线索;阐明
social distancing	社交距离
leak out	漏出;渗出
in terms of	就……而言

1. If the test is _____ , a course of antibiotics may be prescribed.

2. Recent medical studies confirm the _____ of a healthier lifestyle.

3. Some people can have their vision restored by a _____ operation.

4. One _____ of Spanish flu took nearly 22 million lives worldwide.

5. Because of an _____ incompatibility, he is unable to receive a transplant.

6. The packaging must provide an effective _____ to prevent contamination of the product.

7. Heavy drinkers are generally more susceptible to _____ diseases.

8. In the years after the first _____ in the United States, polio was given little attention.

9. Your father is an obvious _____ for a heart attack.

10. Disease of animal and vegetable pests _____ with extreme rapidity.

11. Many skin diseases can be prevented by good personal _____ .

12. The body has natural _____ mechanisms to protect it from disease.

13. It is a report that looks at the medical system from the _____ of deaf people.

14. He dropped a sterile _____ on the floor of the operation room.

15. Heterosexual contact is responsible for the bulk of HIV _____ .

Section B Audio-visual Tasks

Task 2   Spot Dictation

Listen to a passage twice and while listening, you are to put the missing words in each numbered blank according to what you hear.

Medical experts have identified three major kinds of influenza. They call them type A, B and C. Type C is the (1) _____ . People may not even know they have it. But researchers study the other two kinds very closely. Viruses (2) _____ _____ . This can make it difficult for the body to recognize and fight an infection.

Influenza develops after the virus enters a person's nose or mouth. The flu causes (3) _____ , sudden high body temperature, breathing problems and weakness. Generally, most people feel better after a week or two. But the flu can kill. It is especially dangerous to the very young, the very old and those with (4) __ _____ against disease.

A person who has suffered one kind of flu cannot develop that same kind again. The body's defense system (5) _____ . These substances stay in the blood and destroy the virus if it appears again. But the body may not recognize a flu virus that has even a small change.

Researchers (6) _____ a vaccine to protect against bird flu. Still, they know that any vaccine would not be ready until a pandemic had already begun.

Some British researchers say people should be told to wear (7) _____ _____ against infectious diseases, like masks on the face or gloves to protect the hands. The researchers examined fifty-one published studies on the effect of simple ways to prevent (8) _____ infections. They found that hand-washing, wearing masks and using gloves each stopped the (9) _____ . The researchers also found that such physical barriers were even more effective when used together. They said these simple, (10) _____ could prove to be an easy way to prevent the spread of deadly viruses.

Task 3   Short Answer Questions

Listen to the passage "Preventing Flu Pandemic" twice. While listening, you are to give an answer as short as possible to each of the questions below.

1. What do medical experts hope to do when the next outbreak of flu finally happens?

_____

2. What is a pandemic?

_____

3. What is the cause of the Spanish flu pandemic according to the CDC's scientists?

_____

4. When and where did scientists first identify avian influenza?

_____

5. What, according to many researchers, must governments do more to support?

_____

Task 4   Sentence Dictation

Listen to each sentence, repeat it aloud, listen to it again, and then write down the whole sentence in the space provided.

1. _____

   _____

2. _____

   _____

3. _____

   _____

4. _____

   _____

5. _____

   _____

Task 5   Recognizing Details

Watch the video clip "Contact Tracing" twice and decide whether each of the statements below is TRUE (T) *or* FALSE (F).

_____ 1. Without contact tracing, virus transmission among people could get out of control.

_____ 2. Contact tracing is about reaching out to people, calling people who are infected or could be infected and giving them the advice and tools that they need.

_____ 3. Contact tracing is a new method to prevent the transmission of COVID-19.

_____ 4. If you receive a call from a contact tracer, you don't have to take it seriously.

_____ 5. People can be infected with the virus without knowing it.

_____ 6. It is important to find those who have been exposed to the virus and could be infectious.

_____ 7. Contact tracing gives the virus more opportunity to spread in the community.

Task 6   Overall Comprehension

Watch the video clip "Wearing Masks" twice and choose the best answer to each of the questions below.

1. When did masks start to be used to protect the person wearing them?
   A. Around 1918.   B. From the 1990s.
   C. From the 1890s.   D. Right around the 1800s.

2. What are still in high demand for health care professionals?
   A. Welder's shields.   B. Social distancing.
   C. All kinds of masks.   D. Surgical masks and N95s.

3. What are the two most important factors of the efficacy of masks?
   A. The fit and the fabric of masks.
   B. The size and the price of masks.
   C. When and how masks are worn.
   D. Social distancing and hand hygiene.

4. Which of the following statements is NOT true about the new study from UK about masks?
   A. It hasn't been peer reviewed yet.
   B. It found that full-face shields allowed for a strong downward jet.

C. It found that masks decreased the forward momentum of particles by nearly 90%.

D. It found that handmade masks produced jets that can leak out from the sides and the back.

5. Which of the following statements about masks is NOT true?

A. We don't know anything about the efficacy of masks in a lab setting.

B. Wearing masks does not replace social distancing and hand hygiene.

C. We don't know the efficacy of masks at preventing the spread of COVID-19 in real life.

D. We don't know whether the practice of wearing masks would be permanent in the U.S.

Section C   Oral Tasks

Task 7   Listening & Interpretation

Listen to each sentence twice and interpret it into Chinese.

1. _____

   _____

2. _____

   _____

3. _____

   _____

4. _____

   _____

5. _____

   _____

Task 8   Dialogue & Conversation

Make dialogues and conversations, using the Chinese below as cues.

A:随着新冠疫情蔓延,很多人对如此严峻的疫情形势感到恐慌。

B:是呀。新冠病是近百年来人类遭遇的影响范围最广的全球性大流行病。

A：新型冠状病毒可以在人与人之间传播。新型冠状病毒感染后会有哪些主要症状呢？

B：大部分人会出现发热、干咳、乏力、不同程度的呼吸困难等临床症状。

A：那新冠病和普通感冒或流感又有什么区别呢？

B：这些都是呼吸系统疾病，因而临床症状相似，但新冠病传染能力最强、对机体的杀伤力最大。

A：流感疫苗可以降低患流感的风险。我们也应该接种新冠疫苗吗？

B：是的，接种疫苗是疫情防控最经济、最有效的公共卫生干预手段。

A：除了接种疫苗，我们还可以怎样预防新冠病呢？

B：我们还可以通过戴口罩、勤洗手、不去人多的地方来预防新冠病。

A：如果接到疾控部门的接触者追踪电话，我们该怎么办呢？

B：我们应该积极配合调查，帮助阻断病毒的传播。

Task 9   Discussion or Oral Presentation

Discuss briefly in a pair-group or make a 2-minute oral presentation based on the following questions .

1. What are the most common symptoms of influenza?

2. What are the three most important things you have learned about flu prevention?

3. What is contact tracing? Do you think contact tracing is an effective way to prevent epidemics? Why or why not?

4. If you were the university president, how could you encourage students to wear masks properly?

5. What can be done to lower the risk of virus transmission?

Section D   Follow-up Reading

Task 10   Reading Comprehension

Read the passage and complete each statement with a proper phrase or sentence given in the box.

Obviously there is so much attention on wearing masks, including those who choose not to wear one. There is a new study now that sheds some light on the issue.

For some historical perspective, first of all, masks from the 1890s — right around the 1900s — were really used to prevent the spread of infections, just as they're being used now. But around 1918, when we had that big pandemic, they first started to be used to protect the person wearing them. Now we have to remember that masks are just part of PPE (personal protective equipment). Surgical masks and N95s are still in high demand for health care professionals and first responders and their efficacy really depends on the fit and the fabric. So, even though they're all a little bit different, those are the two most important factors, and we have to remember that they do not replace the behaviors like social distancing and hand hygiene.

Now there are all kinds of masks, from makeshift masks to N95s on the street. There's a new study out from the UK about masks on how they work and what the theories are. The results haven't been peer reviewed, but this study from the NHS in the UK looked at all different types of face coverings. The researchers found that, in general, they decreased the forward momentum of particles by at least 90% or more. They also found that those full-face shields that look like the clear welder's kind of shields, did allow a strong downward jet. That's just basic physics. If the air can't go out, it's going to go down. And they looked at handmade masks and found that while they were good at blocking forward momentum of these particles, they did produce jets that could leak out the sides and the back. So it's interesting, in terms of where you might be standing around someone who's wearing one. You might feel very safe behind them, but maybe you aren't. And we need to remember that when you look at something in a lab setting versus real life, you're going to get different results, but we don't know yet efficacy of masks at preventing the spread of COVID-19, and we don't know how effective they are at protecting the person wearing them, because this is really for the protection of others. Will this practice become permanent in the U.S. like it is in many Asian countries? Is this a trend that's here to stay? We just don't know yet. That's all to be determined.

1. We know that right around the 1900s masks were really _____.

2. Even though masks are all a little bit different, their efficacy really _____.

3. A new study from the NHS in the UK found that masks _____.

4. You are going to get different results when you _____.

5. We don't know whether the practice of wearing masks will _____.

A. become permanent in the U.S.

B. depends on the fit and the fabric

C. used to prevent the spread of infections

D. look at something in a lab setting versus real life

E. found the theories of how masks work in different settings

F. decreased the forward momentum of particles by at least 90%

G. make the behaviors like social distancing and hand hygiene unnecessary

Screening and Checkup

Overview

Screening（筛查）, in medicine, is a strategy used to look for as-yet-unrecognied conditions or risk markers. This testing can be applied to individuals or to a whole population. The people tested may not exhibit any signs or symptoms of a disease, or they might exhibit only one or two symptoms, which by themselves do not indicate a definitive diagnosis.

Screening interventions are designed to identify conditions which could at some future point turn into disease, thus enabling earlier intervention and management in the hope to reduce mortality and suffering from a disease.

Several types of screening exist: mass screening, high risk or selective screening, and multiphasic（多相的）screening. Mass screening is the screening of a whole population or subgroup. It is offered to all, irrespective of the risk status of the individual. High risk or selective screening is conducted only among high-risk people. Multiphasic screening refers to the application of two or more screening tests to a large population at one time, instead of carrying out separate screening tests for single diseases.

When done thoughtfully and based on research, identification of risk factors can be a strategy for medical screening.

To many people, screening instinctively seems like an appropriate thing to do, because catching something earlier seems better. However, no screening test is perfect. There will always be the problems with incorrect results. It is an ethical requirement for balanced and accurate information to be given to participants at the point when screening is offered, in order that they can make a fully informed choice about whether or not to accept.

Although screening may lead to an earlier diagnosis, not all screening tests have been shown to benefit the person being screened; overdiagnosis(过度诊断), misdiagnosis(错误诊断), and creating a false sense of security are some potential adverse effects of screening.

Section A　Pre-audio-visual Tasks

Task 1　Glossary Work

Get familiar with the following words and expressions by listening to and reading them. Then match the meaning description or synonym with a proper word or expression in the glossary list.

polyp /ˈpɒlɪp/ *n.*	息肉;珊瑚虫
colonoscopy /ˌkəʊlənəˈskɒpɪ/ *n.*	结肠镜检查(术)
oncologist /ɒŋˈkɒlədʒɪst/ *n.*	肿瘤学家
prevalence /ˈprevələns/ *n.*	(疾病等的)流行程度;盛行
ethnic /ˈeθnɪk/ *adj.*	(少数)民族的;种族的
cervical /ˈsɜːvɪkl/ *adj.*	子宫颈的;颈的
segment /ˈsegmənt/ *n.*	部分;环节
underserved /ʌndəˈsɜːvd/ *adj.*	服务水平低下的;服务不周到的
concerted /kənˈsɜːtɪd/ *adj.*	同心协力的;联合的
osteoporosis /ˌɒstɪəʊpəˈrəʊsɪs/ *n.*	骨质疏松症
pinpoint /ˈpɪnpɔɪnt/ *v.*	确定;准确地指出;精准定位
trait /treɪt/ *n.*	特点;特征
flaw /flɔː/ *n.*	缺点;瑕疵
committed /kəˈmɪtɪd/ *adj.*	坚定的;忠诚的
inspire /ɪnˈspaɪə(r)/ *v.*	激励;启发
grim /grɪm/ *adj.*	严峻的;令人沮丧的
leukemia /luːˈkiːmɪə/ *n.*	白血病
incurable /ɪnˈkjʊərəbl/ *adj.*	无法治愈的;无法改变的

scary /ˈskeərɪ/ *adj.*	使人惊慌的；胆小的
cumulative /ˈkjuːmjələtɪv/ *adj.*	积累的；渐增的
radiation /ˌreɪdɪˈeɪʃn/ *n.*	辐射；放射物
abnormality /ˌæbnɔːˈmælətɪ/ *n.*	变态；畸形；反常
biopsy /ˈbaɪɒpsi/ *n.*	活组织检查
detection /dɪˈtekʃn/ *n.*	发现；察觉
caution /ˈkɔːʃn/ *v.*	提醒；警告
license /ˈlaɪsns/ *n.*	许可证；特许
chest X-ray	胸部 X 线检查
the pros and cons	赞成与反对的理由
Human Genome Project	人类基因组计划
low-dose spiral CT scan	低剂量螺旋 CT 扫描

1. a medical condition in which the bones become brittle and fragile from loss of tissue, typically as a result of hormonal changes, or deficiency of calcium or vitamin D   _____

2. increasing or increased in quantity, degree, or force by successive additions

   _____

3. to say something as a warning   _____

4. the action or process of identifying the presence of something concealed

   _____

5. a malignant progressive disease in which the bone marrow and other blood-forming organs produce increased numbers of immature or abnormal leucocytes

   _____

6. a genetically determined characteristic   _____

7. to fill someone with the urge or ability to do or feel something, especially to do something creative   _____

8. a small growth, usually benign and with a stalk, protruding from a mucous membrane   _____

9. a mark, blemish, or other imperfection which mars a substance or object

   _____

10. to find or identify with great accuracy or precision   _____

11. frightening; causing fear _____

12. a medical practitioner qualified to diagnose and treat tumors _____

13. an examination of tissue removed from a living body to discover the presence, cause, or extent of a disease _____

14. very serious or gloomy _____

15. a procedure in which a flexible fiber-optic instrument is inserted through the anus in order to examine the colon _____

Section B Audio-visual Tasks

Task 2 Spot Dictation

Listen to a conversation twice, and while listening, you are to put the missing words in each numbered blank according to what you hear.

— We're going to talk about screening for — and prevention of — colorectal cancer. Dr. Richardson, is it really possible to prevent colorectal cancer?

— Yes, it is. With the right (1) _____ done at the right time, 60 to 70 percent of colorectal cancers can be prevented with screening. Almost (2) __ _____ between the ages of 50 and 75 have not been screened for colorectal cancer. If we increase the number of people in that group who get screened to 80 or 90 percent, (3) _____ per year will get colorectal cancer altogether.

— Dr. Richardson, explain how screening helps prevent colorectal cancer.

— The screening tests look for (4) _____ called polyps in the lower intestine. Polyps can turn into cancer if they are left untreated. However, if you remove the polyp, the cancer will never happen.

— You said "tests." Is there more than one way to (5) _____ this type of cancer?

— Yes, most people don't know there are a number of tests available. The test people often think about is (6) _____, which is done at a doctor's office. During a colonoscopy, a tube is put into the colon to (7) _____ __. But there are also tests, like stool tests, that people can do at home.

— So why aren't people getting screened?

— Well, there are several reasons. Often, people don't know that they need to be screened. Doctors (8) _____ the test. So ask your doctor if you need to have the test done. And, people are just afraid of cancer.

— You're an oncologist — a cancer doctor — so you've seen people that (9) _____ by colorectal cancer who maybe didn't have to be, if they had gotten screened.

— Yes, and it's not just as a doctor, but as a family member. Colorectal cancer is a tragedy that can often be avoided. My aunt (10) _____ from colorectal cancer that might have been prevented if she had been screened.

Task 3   Note-taking

Listen to the conversation on "Patterns and Trends in Cancer Screening" twice. While listening, you are to take notes according to the cues given below.

1. The research paper mainly reports on:

   _____

2. The use of cancer screening is particularly low in the segments of the population:

   _____

3. One reason why colorectal cancer screening was the only test that increased in use:

   _____

4. Future research is recommended to explore:

   _____

5. Doctors can play a key role in:

   _____

Task 4   Sentence Dictation

Listen to each sentence, repeat it aloud, listen to it again, and then write down the whole sentence in the space provided.

1. _____

   _____

2. _____

3. _____

4. _____

5. _____

Task 5 Recognizing Details

Watch the video clip "Genetic Checkup" twice and decide whether each of the statements below is TRUE (T) *or* FALSE (F).

_____ 1. Malissa Christian is a candidate for marathon runner in spite of her heart disease.

_____ 2. DNA checkup also reveals that Malissa will get diabetes.

_____ 3. Thanks to the Human Genome Project, doctors can now pinpoint genetic traits that might make you sick.

_____ 4. DNA checkup can also identify people who are at risk early in their life for overweight.

_____ 5. A simple blood test cannot check for some genetic flaws that give rise to disease.

_____ 6. Malissa would want to know grim information if a DNA test is offered for incurable diseases.

_____ 7. There are no emotional barriers between patients and DNA technology.

Task 6 Overall Comprehension

Watch the video clip "Lung Cancer Screening" twice and choose the best answer to each of the questions below.

1. What does the new research show?

A. Lung cancer is the number one cancer killer in the U.S.

B. Screening test can be done as a routine test for lung cancer.

C. The number of lung cancer in men and women is significant.

  D. A certain kind of screening test can cut the death rate of lung cancer.

2. Researchers resolved a huge medical controversy with _____ .

  A. the help of reducing the death rate from lung cancer

  B. the study of 53,000 current and former heavy smokers

  C. a screening test of smokers between 55 to 74 years old

  D. a type of screening X-ray called a low-dose spiral CT scan

3. Which of the following statements is NOT true of the participants?

  A. They smoked an average of a pack a day for thirty years.

  B. Some got a low-dose spiral CT scan once a year for three years.

  C. Those who got standard chest X-rays had a better chance of survival.

  D. There were 20 percent fewer deaths among those who got the CT scan.

4. Which of the following is not mentioned as a concern about screening?

  A. Lower efficiency among non-smokers.

  B. Risk of cumulative radiation exposure.

  C. Unnecessary biopsies or surgeries.

  D. A 25 percent false positive rate.

5. Doctors caution that _____ .

  A. non-smokers should get no CT screening

  B. CT scan may cost 300 to 400 dollars

  C. CT scan is not a license to smoke

  D. insurance policies should be changed

Section C Oral Tasks

Task 7 Listening & Interpretation

Listen to each sentence twice and interpret it into Chinese.

1. _____

  _____

2. _____

  _____

3. _____

  _____

4. _____
   _____
5. _____
   _____

Task 8   Dialogue & Conversation

Make dialogues and conversations，using the Chinese below as cues.

A：你了解筛检吗？

B：筛检是在患者出现症状之前对疾病的检测。

A：筛检的目的是什么呢？

B：及早发现慢性病是筛检的目的。

A：你认为筛检有用吗？

B：是的，筛检可以及早发现某些疾病，降低其导致死亡的风险。

A：我需要做哪些筛检呢？

B：这取决于你的年龄、性别、家族史以及你是否存在罹患某些疾病的危险因素。

A：我还是不太确定我是否应该做筛检。

B：别担心。在做筛检之前，和医生探讨一下好处和潜在的危害，以帮助你决定什么对你的健康是最有益的。

Task 9   Discussion or Oral Presentation

Discuss briefly in a pair-group or make a 2-minute oral presentation based on the following questions.

1. What is a screening test in healthcare?
2. What are some common screening tests?
3. What role does a screening test play in cancer prevention?
4. Why are screening tests sometimes controversial?
5. What are the benefits and possible harms of screening tests?

Section D   Follow-up Reading

Task 10   Reading Comprehension

Read the passage and fill in each blank with a proper phrase or sentence given in the box.

New research out tonight shows that a certain kind of scan, when done as a routine test, can cut the death rate and the numbers are significant.

For the first time, researchers have clear evidence that a type of screening x-ray called a low-dose spiral CT scan __1__. The test has been a huge medical controversy for years, but researchers resolved it with the study of 53,000 current and former heavy smokers, fifty-five to seventy-four years old.

"We will be able to pick up early cancer, and if it's picked up there is a chance you will survive this cancer," said Dr. Reginald Munden of M.D. Anderson Cancer Center.

The participants smoked an average of a pack a day for thirty years. The study __2__ to detect lung cancer. Some got a low-dose spiral CT scan once a year for three years. Others got a standard chest X-ray. All were followed for up to another five years. There were 20 percent fewer deaths from lung cancer among those who got the CT scan.

Doctors emphasize the study did not include non-smokers who __3__.

And there are some concerns about risk of cumulative radiation exposure from the CT screening test. Plus, the test also __4__. "But those abnormalities need to be followed up," said Dr. Douglas Lowy of the National Cancer Institute. And that can involve unnecessary biopsy or surgery.

Recommendations about who __5__ could be released within a few months. Doctors say that might influence insurance companies and Medicare to change their policies and cover the scans, which cost 300 to 400 dollars. While doctors say the CT scan is a breakthrough in lung cancer detection, they caution it's not a license to smoke.

_____ 1.

_____ 2.

_____ 3.

_____ 4.

_____ 5.

A. compared the effects of two tests

B. match the tumor to effective drugs

C. should get CT screening for lung cancer

D. produced a 25 percent false positive rate

E. make up 15 percent of lung cancer victims

F. screen the tumors in every single cancer patient

G. can actually help reduce the death rate from lung cancer

Appendix

Glossary

Glossary		Unit
a big chunk of	大量的	3
a big deal	重要的事情	6
a silver lining	一线希望；好的一面	6
abdominal /æb'dɒmɪnl/ *adj*.	腹部的	6
abnormal /æb'nɔːml/ *adj*.	异常的；不正常的	6
abnormality /ˌæbnɔː'mælətɪ/ *n*.	变态；畸形；反常	13
abuse /ə'bjuːs/ *v*.	滥用；虐待；辱骂	7
add up	言之有理；加起来得到理想的结果	1
administer /əd'mɪnɪstə(r)/ *v*.	给予；施行	11
adolescent /ˌædə'lesnt/ *n*.	青少年	7
adopt /ə'dɒpt/ *v*.	采取；收养	3
adrenal gland /ə'drɪːnl glænd/	肾上腺	9
adrenalin /ə'drenəlɪn/ *n*.	肾上腺素	9
aerobic /e'rəʊbɪk/ *adj*.	有氧的；需氧的	4
affect /ə'fekt/ *v*.	影响；感染	3
aggravate /'ægrəveɪt/ *v*.	加重；使恶化	8
aging /'eɪdʒɪŋ/ *n*.	老龄化；老化	4
airway /'erweɪ/ *n*.	(肺的)气道；通气道	11
alcoholism /'ælkəhɒlɪzəm/ *n*.	酗酒	5
all sorts of	各种各样的	3
allergy /'æləːdʒɪ/ *n*.	过敏；过敏性反应	8
Alzheimer's disease /'æltshaɪməz dɪ'ziːz/ *n*.	阿尔茨海默病	2
annoyance /ə'nɔɪəns/ *n*.	恼怒；使人烦恼的事	9
antibody /'æntɪbɒdɪ/ *n*.	抗体	12
antidepressant /ˌæntɪdɪ'presnt/ *n*.	抗抑郁剂	10
anxiety /æŋ'zaɪətɪ/ *n*.	焦虑	6
approach /ə'prəʊtʃ/ *v*.	接近；着手处理	6
apt to	易于	10

cardio /ˈkɑːdɪəʊ/ *adj.*	有氧运动	4
cardiopulmonary /ˌkɑːdɪəʊˈpʌlmənərɪ/ *adj.*	心肺的	11
cardiovascular /ˌkɑːdɪəʊˈvæskjələ(r)/ *adj.*	心血管的	1
category /ˈkætɪgərɪ/ *n.*	种类;部属;类目	11
causal /ˈkɔːzl/ *adj.*	具有因果关系的	5
caution /ˈkɔːʃn/ *v.*	提醒;警告	13
cellphone /ˈselfəʊn/ *n.*	手机	7
ceramic /səˈræmɪk/ *adj.*	陶器的;陶瓷的	8
cervical /ˈsɜːvɪkl/ *adj.*	子宫颈的	6
checklist /ˈtʃeklɪst/ *n.*	清单	10
chest /tʃest/ *n.*	胸部	11
chest X-ray	胸部 X 线检查	13
choking /ˈtʃəʊkɪŋ/ *adj.*	窒息的;憋闷的	11
cholesterol /kəˈlestərɒl/ *n.*	胆固醇	2
chronic /ˈkrɒnɪk/ *adj.*	慢性的;长期的	9
cognitive /ˈkɒgnətɪv/ *adj.*	认知的;认识过程的	7
collapse /kəˈlæps/ *v.*	虚脱	11
colonoscopy /ˌkəʊlənəˈskɒpɪ/ *n.*	结肠镜检查(术)	13
colorectal /ˌkəʊləˈrektəl/ *adj.*	结直肠的	2
come up with	想出;想到	12
committed /kəˈmɪtɪd/ *adj.*	坚定的,忠诚的	13
compelling /kəmˈpelɪŋ/ *adj.*	令人信服的;非常强烈的	4
comprehensive /ˌkɒmprɪˈhensɪv/ *adj.*	全面的;综合性的	5
compression /kəmˈpreʃən/ *n.*	压迫;压缩	11
concerning /kənˈsɜːnɪŋ/ *prep.*	关于;就……而言	3
concerted /kənˈsɜːtɪd/ *adj.*	同心协力的;联合的	13
consequence /ˈkɒnsɪkwens/ *n.*	结果;重要性	3
conservation /ˌkɒnsəˈveɪʃn/ *n.*	保存;保护	8
consistent /kənˈsɪstənt/ *adj.*	一致的;连续的	4
consume /kənˈsjuːm/ *v.*	消费	2
contact tracing	接触者追踪	12
contentious /kənˈtenʃəs/ *adj.*	有争论的	5
conversion /kənˈvɜːʃn/ *n.*	转换;转变	8
cortisol /ˈkɒtɪsɒl/ *n.*	皮质醇;氢化可的松	9
counselor /ˈkaʊnsələ/ *n.*	顾问	10
COVID-19	新型冠状病毒病	12
crusade /kruːˈseɪd/ *n.*	改革运动	2

culprit /ˈkʌlprɪt/ n.	罪犯;肇事者	9
cumulative /ˈkjuːmjələtɪv/ adj.	积累的;渐增的	13
cut short	缩短;剪短;截断	1
cutback /ˈkʌtbæk/ n.	减少;削减	2
debate /dɪˈbeɪt/ n.	争论;辩论;讨论	4
defense /dɪˈfens/ n.	防御能力;防御;辩护	12
define /dɪˈfaɪn/ v.	界定;下定义	4
deliberate /dɪˈlɪbərət/ adj.	蓄意的;小心翼翼的	1
delicate /ˈdelɪkət/ adj.	微妙的;精致的;脆弱的	9
delivery business	运输;快递业	3
depressed /dɪˈprest/ adj.	抑郁的;沮丧的	10
depression /dɪˈpreʃn/ n.	沮丧;抑郁;萎靡不振	4
detection /dɪˈtekʃn/ n.	发现;察觉	13
diabetes /ˌdaɪəˈbiːtiːz/ n.	糖尿病	1
diagnose /ˌdaɪəgˈnəʊs/ v.	诊断;判断	7
dietary /ˈdaɪətəri/ adj.	饮食的;规定饮食的	2
dieter /ˈdaɪətə(r)/ n.	(旨在减肥的)节食者	5
digestive system	消化系统	2
disability /ˌdɪsəˈbɪləti/ n.	残疾;无能	1
disconcerting /ˌdɪskənˈsɜːtɪŋ/ adj.	令人不安的	6
dismal /ˈdɪzməl/ adj.	凄凉的;悲惨的	6
disorder /dɪsˈɔːdər/ n.	(身心)失调;不适;病	1
distract /dɪˈstrækt/ v.	分散(注意力);使分心	7
divorced /dɪˈvɔːst/ adj.	离婚的	10
dramatically /drəˈmætɪkli/ adv.	显著地;引人注目地	3
drown /draʊn/ v.	(使)淹死;淹没	11
dysregulation /dɪːzregjʊˈleɪʃn/ n.	失调	3
ease /iːz/ v.	减轻;缓解	9
ecosystem /ˈiːkəʊsɪstəm/ n.	生态系统	8
effectiveness /ɪˈfekˈtɪvnɪs/ n.	效力	3
efficacy /ˈefɪkəsi/ n.	功效;效力;效验	12
electrocution /ɪˌlektrəˈkjuːʃn/ n.	电击;电死	11
emergency /iˈmɜːdʒənsi/ n.	紧急;急症;意外	11
emotion /ɪˈməʊʃn/ n.	情感;情绪	3
emphasize /ˈemfəsaɪz/ v.	强调;重视	11
endorphin /enˈdɔːfɪn/ n.	内啡肽(体内产生有镇痛作用的激素)	4
enhance /ɪnˈhæns/ v.	提高;增强	4

equation /ɪˈkweɪʒn/ *n*.	等式;平衡	5
esthetic /iːsˈθetɪk/ *adj*.	美学的;审美的	8
ethical /ˈeθɪkl/ *adj*.	伦理的;道德的	8
ethnic /ˈeθnɪk/ *adj*.	(少数)民族;种族的	13
evaluate /ɪˈvæljʊeɪt/ *v*.	评价;估价	4
eventually /ɪˈventʃʊəlɪ/ *adv*.	最后;终于	6
exhaustion /ɪgˈzɔːstʃən/ *n*.	精疲力竭;耗尽	3
expel /ɪkˈspel/ *v*.	呼出空气;排出	11
fabric /ˈfæbrɪk/ *n*.	织物;结构	12
faint /feɪnt/ *v*.	昏晕;昏倒	11
fatty acid	脂肪酸	2
fetus /ˈfiːtəs/ *n*.	胎儿	2
fidget /ˈfɪdʒɪt/ *v*.	坐立不安;烦躁	5
fight-or-flight response	战或逃反应	9
Finland /ˈfɪnlənd/ *n*.	芬兰	7
first aid	急救	11
flaw /flɔː/ *n*.	缺点;瑕疵	13
folic acid	叶酸	2
formaldehyde /fɔːˈmældɪhaɪd/ *n*.	甲醛	8
friction /ˈfrɪkʃn/ *n*.	摩擦;摩擦力;冲突;不和	1
genetics /dʒəˈnetɪks/ *n*.	遗传学	9
get out of control	失去控制	12
glove /glʌv/ *n*.	手套	12
grief-stricken /ˈgriːf ˈstrɪkən/ *adj*.	极度忧伤的	10
grieve /griːv/ *v*.	使伤心;使悲伤	10
grim /grɪm/ *adj*.	严峻的;令人沮丧的	13
guarantee /gærənˈtiː/ *v*.	保证;担保	6
guilty /ˈgɪltɪ/ *adj*.	内疚的;有罪的	8
hardship /ˈhɑːdʃɪp/ *n*.	艰苦	10
heart attack	心脏病发作	11
heighten /ˈhaɪtn/ *v*.	提高;加强	9
herring /ˈherɪŋ/ *n*.	鲱鱼	2
homocystine /həʊməʊˈsɪstiːn/ *n*.	高胱氨酸	2
hormone therapy	激素疗法	6
Human Genome Project	人类基因组计划	13
humidity /hjuːˈmɪdətɪ/ *n*.	湿度;潮湿	8
hygiene /ˈhaɪdʒiːn/ *n*.	卫生;卫生学	12

life expectancy	期望寿命，平均寿命	1
lifting weight	举重	4
locale /ləʊˈkɑːl/ *n*.	场所或地点	1
low-dose spiral CT scan	低剂量螺旋 CT 扫描	13
lycopene /ˈlaɪkəpiːn/ *n*.	番茄红素	2
mackerel /ˈmækrəl/ *n*.	鲭鱼	2
magic bullet	灵丹妙药;妙招	5
mammogram /ˈmæməgræm/ *n*.	乳腺 X 线片	6
mannequin /ˈmænɪkɪn/ *n*.	人体模型	11
max /mæks/ *adj*.	最高的;最多的	9
medicate /ˈmedɪkeɪt/ *v*.	用药医治	7
medication /ˌmedɪˈkeɪʃn/ *n*.	药物，药剂;药物治疗	1
meditation /ˌmedɪˈteɪʃn/ *n*.	沉思;冥想	9
Mediterranean diet	地中海饮食	2
medium /ˈmiːdɪəm/ *adj*.	中等的;平均的	4
misdiagnose /mɪsˈdaɪəgnəʊz/ *v*.	误诊	10
mistakenly /mɪˈsteɪkənlɪ/ *adv*.	错误地;曲解地	3
mobilize /ˈməʊbəlaɪz/ *v*.	动员;组织	9
moderate /ˈmɒdərət, ˈmɒdəreɪt/ *adj*.	适度的	5
modification /mɒdɪfɪˈkeɪʃn/ *n*.	改变;变形;变更;修正	1
moody /ˈmuːdɪ/ *adj*.	喜怒无常的	10
morality /məˈrælətɪ/ *n*.	道德;道德准则;道德观	7
motivate /ˈməʊtɪveɪt/ *v*.	驱使;激发……的兴趣	9
multitasking /ˌmʌltɪˈtæskɪŋ/ *n*.	多(重)任务处理	7
nightmare /ˈnaɪtmeə/ *n*.	噩梦;梦魇	6
nitrogen oxide /ˈnaɪtrədʒən ˈɒksaɪd/ *n*.	氧化氮	8
nugget /ˈnʌgɪt/ *n*.	一条(信息);块状物	5
nutritious /njʊˈtrɪʃəs/ *adj*.	有营养的;滋养的	5
oat /əʊt/ *n*.	燕麦;麦片粥	2
obesity /əʊˈbiːsɪtɪ/ *n*.	肥胖，肥胖症	1
obligation /ˌɒblɪˈgeɪʃn/ *n*.	义务;责任	9
on the go	忙忙碌碌的;不停奔走的	6
oncologist /ɒŋˈkɒlədʒɪst/ *n*.	肿瘤学家	13
onset /ˈɒnset/ *n*.	发病;开始;攻击	7
Ornish /ˈɔːnɪʃ/ *n*.	欧尼许(饮食法)	5
osteoporosis /ˌɒstɪəʊpəˈrəʊsɪs/ *n*.	骨质疏松症	13
outbreak /ˈaʊtbreɪk/ *n*.	(战争、疾病等的)爆发;突然发生	12

psychological /ˌsaɪkəˈlɒdʒɪkl/ *adj*.	心理的;精神上的	4
psychologist /saɪˈkɒlədʒɪst/ *n*.	心理学家	9
puberty /ˈpjuːbərtɪ/ *n*.	青春期,发育期;开花期	7
push-up /pʊʃ ʌp/ *n*.	俯卧撑	4
put sth. on the back burner	把……搁置	6
radiation /ˌreɪdɪˈeɪʃn/ *n*.	辐射;放射物	13
reach out to	联系;把手伸向	12
recession /rɪˈseʃn/ *n*.	衰退;不景气	6
recovery /rɪˈkʌvərɪ/ *n*.	(身体的)恢复;康复	10
red flag	危险信号	6
regain /rɪˈgeɪn/ *v*.	恢复;重回;复得	5
regardless of	不管;不顾	4
reinforce /ˌriːɪnˈfɔːs/ *v*.	加强	1
release /rɪˈliːs/ *v*.	释放;公布	4
relief /rɪˈliːf/ *n*.	减轻;宽慰;解脱	3
reluctant /rɪˈlʌktənt/ *adj*.	不情愿的;厌恶的	11
repetitive /rɪˈpetətɪv/ *adj*.	重复的;反复的	7
rescue /ˈreskjuː/ *n*.	援救;营救	11
resource /rɪˈsɔːs/ *n*.	资源;物力	10
respond /rɪˈspɒnd/ *v*.	回答;回应;作出反应	7
responder /rɪˈspɒndə/ *n*.	回应者;响应器	12
resume /rɪˈzuːm/ *v*.	重新开始;重返	11
resuscitation /rɪˌsʌsɪˈteɪʃn/ *n*.	复苏	11
revealing /rɪˈviːlɪŋ/ *adj*.	揭露真相的;(服装)暴露的	4
rib /rɪb/ *n*.	肋骨	11
rinse /rɪns/ *v*.	冲洗;冲掉	1
saliva /səˈlaɪvə/ *n*.	唾液,口水	9
salmon /ˈsæmən/ *n*.	鲑鱼,大马哈鱼	2
saturated /ˈsætʃəreɪtɪd/ *adj*.	饱和的	2
scan /skæn/ *v*.	扫描;浏览;细看	7
scary /ˈskeərɪ/ *adj*.	使人惊慌的;胆小的	13
screening /ˈskriːnɪŋ/ *n*.	筛查	6
sedentary /ˈsednterɪ/ *adj*.	久坐不活动的	1
seek treatment	就医	10
segment /ˈsegmənt/ *n*.	部分;环节	13
serving /ˈsɜːvɪŋ/ *n*.	一人份	2
severity /sɪˈverətɪ/ *n*.	严重;严格;严谨	7

the pros and cons	赞成与反对的理由	13
the spinal cord	脊髓	11
The Zone /ðəzəʊn/ *n*.	区域饮食法	5
tiredness /ˈtaɪədnəs/ *n*.	疲劳，疲倦	3
trait /treɪt/ *n*.	特点；特征	13
trans fat	反式脂肪	2
transmission /trænzˈmɪʃn/ *n*.	传播；传送	12
transportation /ˌtrænspɔːˈteɪʃn/ *n*.	运输	3
trauma /ˈtrɔːmə/ *n*.	创伤；外伤	10
trigger /ˈtrɪɡə(r)/ *v*.	引发；触发	9
unavoidable /ˌʌnəˈvɔɪdəbl/ *adj*.	不可避免的	9
uncomplicated /ʌnˈkɒmplɪkeɪtɪd/ *adj*.	简单的；不复杂的	11
uncontrollable /ˌʌnkənˈtrəʊləbl/ *adj*.	难以控制的	9
underserved /ʌndəˈsɜːvd/ *adj*.	服务水平低下的；服务不周到的	13
unprecedented /ʌnˈpresɪdentɪd/ *adj*.	前所未有的；空前的	10
unsatisfactory /ʌnˌsætɪsˈfæktərɪ/ *adj*.	令人不满意的	6
urge /ɜːdʒ/ *v*.	催促；驱使	3
urination /jʊərɪˈneɪʃn/ *n*.	排尿	6
variability /verɪəˈbɪlətɪ/ *n*.	可变性；易变性	2
villain /ˈvɪlən/ *n*.	坏人，恶棍，罪犯	2
volatile /ˈvɒlətaɪl/ *adj*.	易变的；不稳定的；易挥发的	8
voracious /vəˈreɪʃəs/ *adj*.	贪吃的；贪婪的	5
vulnerable /ˈvʌlnərəbl/ *adj*.	易患病的；易受伤的	8
wage /weɪdʒ/ *v*.	进行；开展	3
waist-hip /weɪst hɪp/ *adj*.	腰臀的	1
whopping /ˈwɒpɪŋ/ *a*.	不平常的；巨大的；庞大的	1
wiggle /ˈwɪɡl/ *v*.	摆动；扭动	5
work out	锻炼；解决；进展顺利	4

图书在版编目(CIP)数据

当代医学英语视听说教程. I, 健康促进/陈社胜总主编; 黎亮, 杨克西, 李艳主编. —2 版.
—上海: 复旦大学出版社, 2023.4
(复旦博学. 当代医学英语系列)
ISBN 978-7-309-16696-5

I.①当… Ⅱ.①陈… ②黎… ③杨… ④李… Ⅲ.①医学-英语-听说教学-高等学校-教材
Ⅳ.①R

中国国家版本馆 CIP 数据核字(2023)第 015022 号

当代医学英语视听说教程 I ——健康促进(第 2 版)
陈社胜 总主编 黎 亮 杨克西 李 艳 主编
责任编辑/贺 琦 庄彩云

复旦大学出版社有限公司出版发行
上海市国权路 579 号 邮编: 200433
网址: fupnet@ fudanpress.com http://www.fudanpress.com
门市零售: 86-21-65102580 团体订购: 86-21-65104505
出版部电话: 86-21-65642845
上海华业装潢印刷厂有限公司

开本 787 × 1092 1/16 印张 9.25 字数 165 千
2023 年 4 月第 2 版
2023 年 4 月第 2 版第 1 次印刷

ISBN 978-7-309-16696-5/R · 2023
定价: 60.00 元